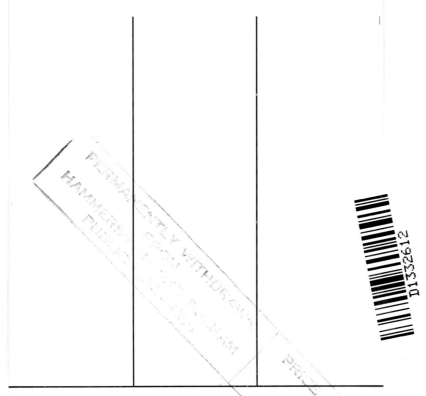
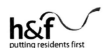

TO MY MUM, WHO WENT THE DISTANCE, every day, every month, every year.

ACKNOWLEDGMENTS

I would like to thank the following people: Frankie Pryor, Les Clark, Pat Orr, Paul Speak, Bernard Micallef, Margaretha Olschewski, and Doris Hartwich for the fantastic photos of the world champions.

I would like to say a special thank-you to "Young" Ernie McQuillan, who took the photos of me in training. Thanks also to Emmanuel Steward, Cheryl McCullough, Ray Wheatley, Jim "The Pehman" Smith, Victor Grynberg of Lonsdale, Steven Dellar, Brian and Robyn at Zoe's boxing shop, and the late, great George Francis. RIP.

To all the team at ABC Books: Jill Brown, Helen Cooney, Steve Collins and Nicola Young. Thanks for making my dream come true.

Thank you to all the fantastic members of the boxing fraternity that I've met on my travels around the world; and to the boxers, trainers, promoters and boxing fans.

To the world champions in this book. Thanks for being part of this project and for the unforgettable memories.

To my wife Jenny and my three kids, John, Erin and Hannah. You were, and always will be, my inspiration. I love you to my heart.

Picture Credits: Jeff Fenech/Ernie McQuillan; Jeff Harding/Ernie McQuillan; Kostya Tszyu/Pat Roth, Fightphotos (p. 26) and the Daily Telegraph, (p. 29); Nigel Benn/Les Clark, Boxpics; Wayne McCullough/Getty Images; Roy Jones Junior/Pat Orr; Fernando Vargas/Pat Orr; Muhammad Ali/Lonsdale (p. 55) and Getty Images (p. 56); Leon Spinks/Getty Images; Ricardo Lopez/Pat Orr; Sven Ottke/Margaretha Olschewski and Doris Hartwich; Ricky Hatton/Paul Speak; Aaron Pryor/Frankie Pryor; Iran Barkley/Getty Images; Livingstone Bramble/Pat Orr; Juan LaPorte/Ernie McQuillan; Donald Curry/Getty Images; Terry Norris/Getty Images; Mike McCallum/Les Clark, Boxpics; Christy Martin/Pat Orr; Frank Bruno/Getty Images; Charlie Magri/Bernard Micallef; Chris Byrd/Pat Orr

Every effort has been made to trace the original source for the pictures contained in this book. Please contact the publisher in the case of any omission.

Published in the U.S. by
Ulysses Press
P.O. Box 3440
Berkeley CA 94703
www.ulyssespress.com

First published as Boxing's Greatest Workouts in Australia in 2005 by ABC Books

Interior designed by Steve Collins @ bingosmithdesign
Cover designed by Jake Flaherty
Front cover photo courtesy of Lonsdale London
Back cover photo © Pat Orr

Printed in Canada by Webcom

10 9 8 7 6

ISBN 978-1-56975-443-6
Library of Congress Control Number 2004108866

Distributed by Publishers Group West

Workouts
from
Boxing's
Greatest
Champs

Including
Muhammad Ali,
Roy Jones, Jr.
Fernando Vargas
and Other Legends

Gary Todd

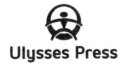

Ulysses Press

CONTENTS

Fighting words 7

A typical day in the life of a champ 16

Jeff Fenech Jeff Harding Kostya Tszyu Nigel Benn Ken Buchanan Wayne McCullough

Roy Jones Junior Glenn Catley Fernando Vargas Ken Norton Muhammad Ali Leon Spinks

Ricardo Lopez Sven Ottke Ricky Hatton Aaron Pryor Iran Barkley Livingstone Bramble

Juan LaPorte Donald Curry Terry Norris Matthew Saad Muhammad Mike McCallum

Christy Martin Frank Bruno Charlie Magri Chris Byrd

My workout 112

Action plan 114

My program 132

When i met... 140

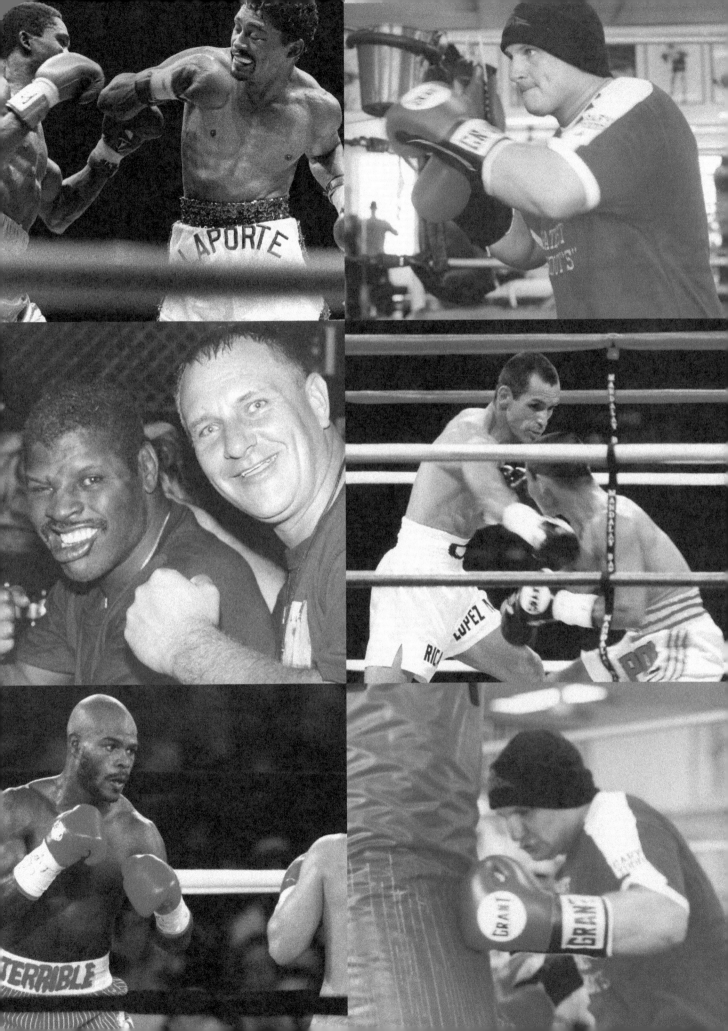

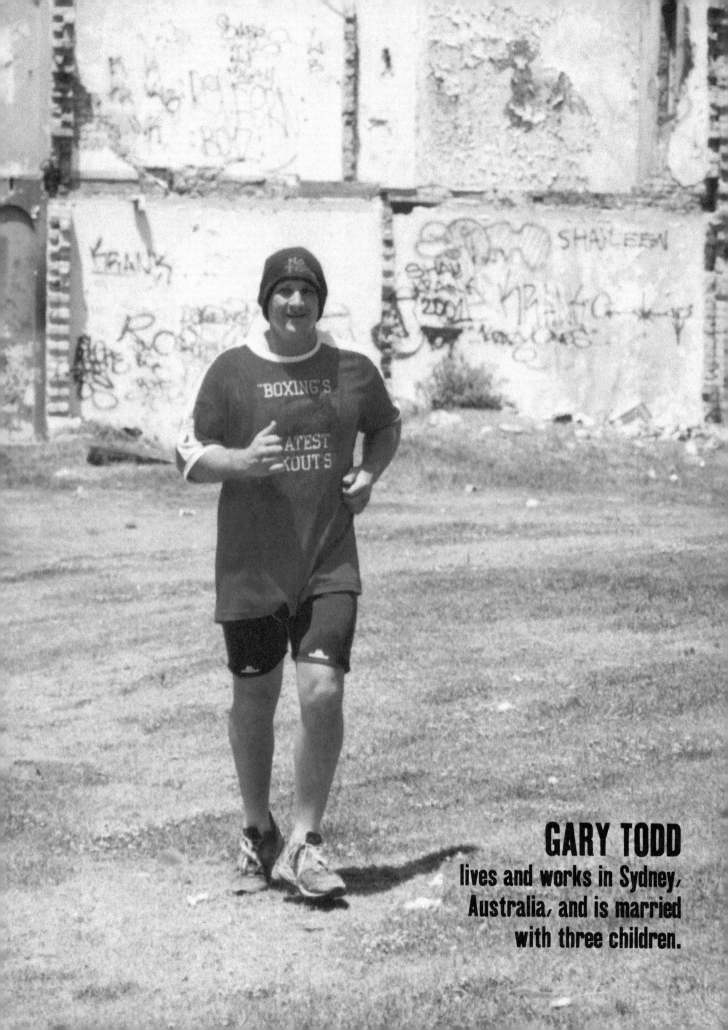

GARY TODD
lives and works in Sydney,
Australia, and is married
with three children.

FiGHTiNG WORDS

You never forget the smell of a boxing gym. It's an overwhelming mixture of sweat, liniment, IcyHot and more sweat. I love walking into a gym, soaking up the atmosphere, seeing everyone busy, the young kids trying their hearts out. You hear the swooshing of the skipping rope, the "di-da-di-di-da-di" of the speed bag, the shouts of the trainers, the pounding of gloves on body and leather. These are the ingredients of a good working gym. And no matter where you go in the world, from Rangoon to Rio, from Rhode Island to Randwick Junction, you'll experience that same atmosphere and see athletes striving to improve. For me, it's a magic place.

The greatest boxing champions of all time — legends like Muhammad Ali and Jeff Fenech, warriors like Kostya Tszyu and Nigel Benn, artisans like Roy Jones Junior — all emerged from gyms just like these. They followed their workouts, sweated and strived, they pushed themselves to the limit to achieve their goals. In the process they felt the incredible high that comes from pitting yourself against yourself. They grew in confidence, they earned the respect of their peers and they felt pride in their achievements.

And they became as fit as men can be.

DO iT

It's no secret that dragging yourself out of bed early in the morning isn't fun, especially when it's dark, cold or raining (or in my case growing up, snowing). So how did these men overcome the everyday hurdles of life? Well, here's the tip: that morning view out the window is the same for anyone, world champions included. They're human, but they've found ways and means to get themselves out of bed, ways to motivate

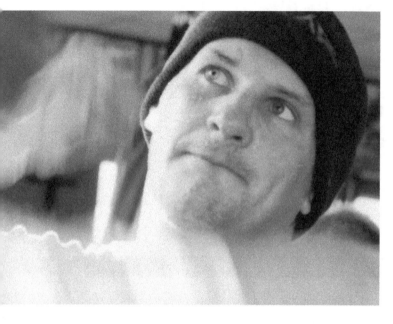

SURViVE iT

I grew up in a sprawling, multistory housing estate in Dundee. It's a small city of about 250,000, but to me it was huge. Life there could be tough. When I was about 11 years old, I noticed a lot of changes taking place. I started watching violent videos at my friend's house when his parents were out. I saw some of my friends joining gangs and starting to sniff glue. I remember the first time I saw two gangs fighting. I was in my kitchen and heard this

iT WAS LiKE A SCENE FROM THE MOViE *BRAVEHEART* . . .
Grown men, teenagers and kids,
ALL CARRYiNG STiCKS AND ROCKS, RUNNiNG TOWARD EACH OTHER

themselves to press on when things were tough — for just getting out and doing it.

When I interviewed the boxers for this book, I asked them what kept them going, what motivated them. They all gave the same, bluntly honest answer — money! When I asked them what enthused them as kids in the amateur ranks, they all said — prizes, medals and trophies. That's why they are often called "prizefighters": that is their major motivation.

But we're all different. We all have different motivations and goals. Mine have their roots in the unforgiving streets of a Scottish city.

roar from outside. I went over to the window and couldn't believe what I was seeing. It was like a scene from the movie *Braveheart*. There were grown men, teenagers and young kids, all carrying sticks and rocks, running toward each other. It was crazy. I noticed they had different-colored jerseys on, so that they could tell the gangs apart. Later, I found out a lady in our block had taken so many orders to make the different gang jerseys that she'd given up her daytime job at the factory. I also remember a guy who came into our area wearing the "wrong" color jersey. He was chased down and kicked so badly that he lost his eye. He was only a young guy and I couldn't believe that something like that could happen in my area.

It was about then I thought: *this is not for me*. I wanted a different future. I especially thought of my mom. I felt she'd had enough heartache in her life without me getting into gang warfare. This was a major reason for dedicating my life to something better. I was going to train to be fit and healthy. I was going to escape the violence. I was going to move on and make something of my life.

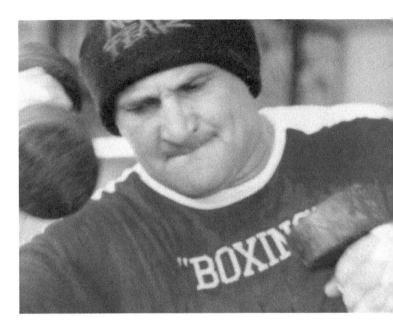

When I was 12, I joined the local community center and got into weight training. Immediately it gave me a real kick. Training soon became the major focus in life, my goal to be the best I could be, to make people — myself included — proud. Around the same time, the movie *Rocky* was on at my local theater. I'll never forget coming out of the theater, jumping around trying to shadowbox, shouting "*Adriennnnne!*" and trying to talk like Stallone. I know it sounds crazy, but that film really motivated me to train and get fit. Even now, when I go on my road-work training runs, I always listen to the *Rocky* theme to help me get going.

I'll also never forget when I first decided to join a boxing club. My friend Eck also wanted to join, so we arranged to meet and go together. It was a bit of a hike but we were eager to make the journey. To get there we had to get on a bus, then get off and walk about two miles through a spooky old railway line that led up to the main road where the gym was. It was pitch black, so we'd scare the shit out of each other as we ran along. It was great fun. When we got to the gym, an old guy threw smelly boxing gloves at us and said, "Get these on." I couldn't believe it — ten minutes before I'd been goofing around with my friend Eck, now I had to fight him! Both of us jumped through the ropes and onto the padded floor. It felt like the loneliest place in the world. We didn't know how to throw a decent punch between us, but somehow we managed to get through it. The old guy came over to us and said, "Well done." We'd got in!

I loved training and mingling with the boxers and the old trainers, listening to their stories. They were all characters and I'll never forget them. They'd sit swigging from their hip flasks, exchanging stories about the old days. But every now and then you'd hear, "Move yer head, son" or "On yer toes, on yer toes."

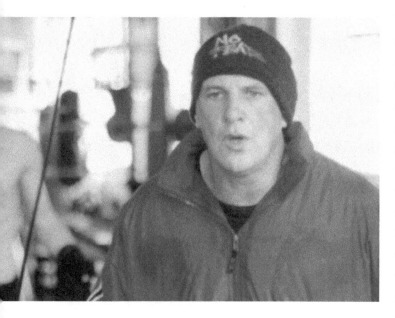

MOVE iT

The years passed and I had left school early to try and make some money for me and my mom. I have no regrets about doing this — I wasn't that enthusiastic about school, although it did give me a good background in reading and writing, which has since helped me in my professional career in the construction industry. I kept up the training and started adding a fair bit of running roadwork. I began by running to and from work. Later, I would go out at night and run a slow five miles and build up my speed as I progressed. I usually finished my run with some hill sprints up the Timex Brae, a Dundee landmark. It was 500 meters from bottom to top and I used to pump my legs up that hill! When I reached the top, all I thought of was Rocky running up the stairs in Philadelphia, and I would punch the air when I got there. A few months later,

I met a guy named Macko while I was out running and we decided to train together. He was a great lad and a great distance runner. One night we were out on a long run in the country when he suddenly pulled out this little tube and started to put it into his mouth. I said, "What the fuck's that?" He told me he was an asthmatic and he needed this now and then to keep him going. He had a little puff and he was away again. This was a great motivator for me — I wasn't going to let a wheezy bastard get the better of me! Macko was a good friend. He always brought out the best in me, especially on our long runs out in the freezing cold hills of Dundee. We started by doing five to seven miles, four times a week and worked up to eleven miles, five nights a week, as well as a long run on a Sunday. We must have run thousands of miles together and we completed many marathons along the way.

CHANGE iT

By 1986 things in Scotland weren't getting any better. Margaret Thatcher had fucked up the working man and there wasn't much left for me there. A friend of mine asked me if I would like to go to Australia with him and I didn't hesitate. We had to save for our big move Down Under. I started working at night in a deer factory, where my job was skinning the deer carcasses and cutting them up into sections for the butchers. The money was good and it helped me achieve my goal. Nine months later we were on our way to Oz.

When we arrived and settled into our new way of life, I got back into my training. I found a brilliant gym that was right on the beach. It was a great place to train and I made a lot of new friends. There were bodybuilders, rugby players, boxers and even ballet dancers training there. I met a few boxers who gave me all the information on the boxing scene in Sydney. I started to float around the gyms and train, much like I do today. At the time, the interest in boxing was

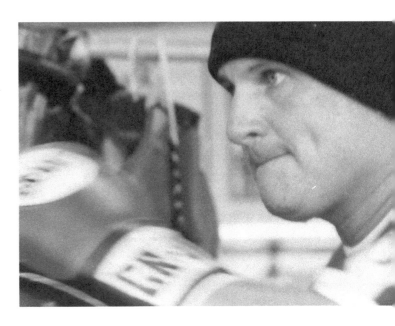

i FOUND A BRiLLiANT GYM THAT WAS RiGHT ON THE BEACH
it was a great place to train
AND i MADE A LOT OF NEW FRiENDS

quite big, as Jeff Fenech had just won the world title. There was also an up-and-coming tough guy named Jeff Harding. It was an exciting time for Australian boxing fans and for the kids in the gyms who dreamed of capturing a world crown for themselves.

LiVE iT

Since getting involved in the Australian boxing scene, I've been in the ring sparring with world champs and have joked with them afterward. I've had a ball. One of my favorite memories is when I traveled to the United States on a boxing trip. I went across to New York

to see the Lewis versus Holyfield title fight at Madison Square Garden. The afternoon of the fight I went down to Brooklyn to do a bit of training with the locals — something I always do when I go overseas. This is often the best part, going to these famous gyms and training with up-and-coming "hungry" fighters. I eventually got to the door of the gym and spoke to the guy in the front office for a little while. He asked me where I was from and if I wanted to box. I said I'd just like to punch the bags and do a bit of jumping rope. When I asked him where the heavy bags were, he said to me in his thick New York accent, "Scottie, I've got the

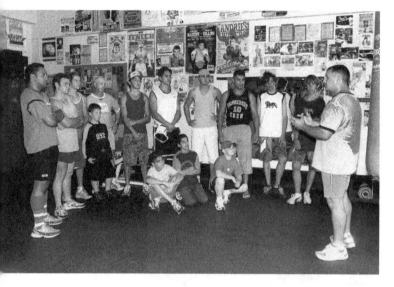

I was nervous, but I continued to get ready while he finished his burger. When he finally got geared up and did his warm-up, he jumped in the ring, walked over and looked down at me; he smiled and then thumped my 18-ounce gloves. At that moment I thought back to my old pal Rocky, when he fought Thunderlips in *Rocky III*.

The buzzer sounded for the first round. We moved out into the center of the ring and I jabbed out — to my surprise, I was snapping his head back.

i WANT TO KEEP THESE KiDS OUT OF TROUBLE
i want to keep them active
i WANT TO SEE THEM GO ON TO BiGGER AND BETTER THiNGS

biggest mother-fucking bag in town." He got on the phone and shouted down it, "Jack, Jack, get your big ass down here!" I jumped into the conversation and said, "Whoa, wait a minute, I'm only here to train, mate!" I was (to say the least) a bit nervous at the thought of "Big Jack" punching the shit out of me, but I was there and I would have looked a bit crazy leaving. So there were only two ways out: either on my back or walking out with my pride intact. I started to get warmed up with some stretching and shadowboxing when the door suddenly opened and this guy appeared. He came through the door sideways, eating a cheeseburger. I couldn't believe the size of this guy. He was big, all right.

He then started his own rally and caught me with a cracker under the ribs, so I grabbed him and finished strong as the round came to an end: Round No.1 to the Scotsman! *Bzzzzz*, and we're away again. The second round was a good one for the big fella and he was continually leaning on me and trying to tire me out, but I was still doing not too bad. The round ended and I thought to myself, "Only two to go." When we came out for the third, he came running over and I managed to duck under his hook and land a big punch to his jaw. He mumbled something at me and threw a haymaker. It connected with the side of my head and it felt like I was flying all the way across to the corner post. My wee legs held out though, and I stayed up. As luck had it, just as he came over to give me some more, the buzzer sounded.

Although I was a bit fuzzy, I knew it was one to go and that I'd taken his best. Now it was time to take a chance and open up for the last round. *Bzzzzz*, we touched gloves and punched the shit out of each other for three minutes. At the end he gave me a cuddle and sort of smiled. I was spent, but very happy. Later on, we had a chat and I asked for a photo so I could show the family when I got home. When I got back to Sydney, I showed my wife — she looked at the photo, looked at me, looked again at the photo, and then walked away, shaking her head, saying nothing.

Anyway, the next morning I woke up and my body was aching all over. I shuffled into the shower and got dressed before making my way down to breakfast in the hotel café. To get into the café you had to go outside to an entrance on the corner. It was snowing. I stepped out onto the cold street. As I reached the door, I pulled out my wallet to check my funds. A single twenty-dollar bill fell out and drifted down to the snow-covered pavement below. I looked around. I tried to bend over to pick up the twenty bucks, but I just couldn't manage it. My bravado with "Big Jack" had taken its toll. I had to leave it there on the snow and hope someone who really needed it would pick it up. But hey, twenty dollars for a memory like that — too cheap!

These days I do a bit of corner work, which means I give boxers instructions and generally look after them during a fight. I continue to train as hard as I can. By far the most satisfying work is helping out with a group of kids, ranging in age from about ten upward. Most are from working-class backgrounds and they just need a bit of guidance. Apart from the physical training, I try to guide them through good and bad experiences. I tell them about my friends on the glue back home and what they are like now. I want to keep them out of trouble, keep these kids active and focused, and hopefully see them go on to bigger and better things. If I can achieve this, then I'll feel I've given something worthwhile back to the sport that I love.

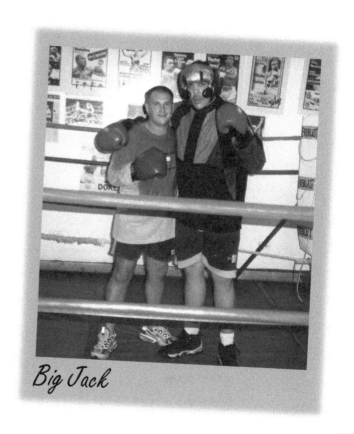

Big Jack

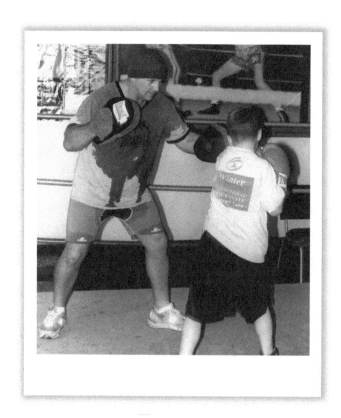
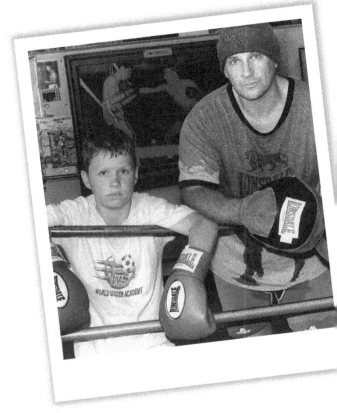

i WiLL ALWAYS TRAiN AS HARD AS MY BODY LETS ME
if you look after your body
YOUR BODY WiLL LOOK AFTER YOU iN YOUR OLD AGE

TRY iT

In life, I believe that as long as you use common sense, you're well-mannered and straight with people, and you live with your morals intact, that's all you need. I once wrote down what motivates me to stick with my training, and it's still true today:

- **personal well-being (mind and body fitness)**
- **self-esteem**
- **pride**
- **confidence**
- **family**
- **medals and trophies**

These are the things you can take from boxing training. These are things that can make a real difference in your life.

And while we can't all be world champs, you can still train like one. This book contains 27 world-class workouts you can do any time of the day. Choose a particular boxer's workout, follow it and build on it until you feel like having a crack at someone else. Maybe you could have six weeks following Kostya Tszyu's workout, followed by a month of Leon Spinks's.

I've tried them all, and let me tell you: you'll never feel fitter.

Because I know how difficult it is to race from work to catch a fitness class, I've also

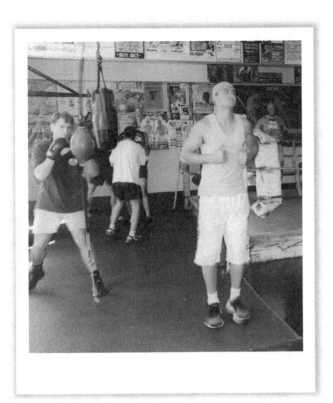

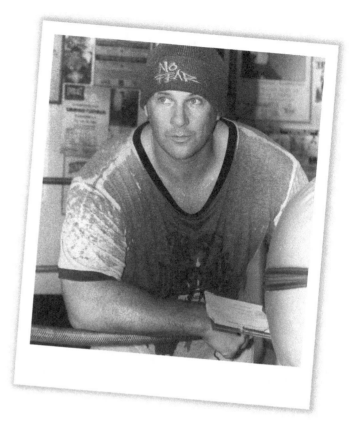

included my own workout, with a guide on how to combine various aspects of my training into your own regimen. This way you can complete a brilliant, all-around workout when you've got time to do it. It's tailored to different fitness levels, so you won't get stuck in a rut. And you'll always have a fitness goal — something to work toward to be the best you can be.

The most important things in my life are my wife and family (whom I love more than I can tell you on paper), my work and, of course, boxing. We all have our commitments — these are mine. I'm a self-confessed boxaholic and I will always train as hard as my body lets me. I'm a great believer that if you look after your body through life, then your body will respond favorably in old age.

I hope this book allows you to experience the very real natural highs you can get from boxing training. I hope you're able to feel firsthand what the champions went through. I hope that when you're struggling toward your hundredth sit-up of the day you can empathize with Fenech or Tszyu or the great Ali, and you can push yourself by thinking about what can be achieved through old-fashioned blood, sweat and tears.

The champions within these pages might say they're motivated by money or titles, but on their individual journeys they were given so much more. They earned self-confidence, self-respect and superb fitness, both mental and physical. In short, they were ordinary men living extraordinary lives, but it was in the boxing gyms that they honed their bodies and minds. Now, I hope, you can too.

Please, enjoy the read.

A TYPICAL
DAY IN THE LIFE

CHA

CHAMP

OF A

MP

JEFF FENECH

What time did you get up?
5:00 a.m.

Did you stretch before your run?
No, never

How far did you run?
3–5 miles, cross-country

What did you do after your run?
Sit-ups in sets of 20 until i reached 200, then i did 15 minutes on the StairMaster. i then had a shower and went to bed.

What did you eat for breakfast?
Porridge and fruit

What did you do after breakfast?
Relaxed, and i always watched *Days of Our Lives*

What time did you go to the gym?
2:00 p.m.

What time did you leave the gym?
4:00 p.m.

What did you do after training?
Rested my body, then had dinner at 5:30 p.m.

What did you eat for dinner?
Steamed veggies and chicken (no red meat)

What did you do after dinner?
Watched TV, went for a walk, and i liked to read

What time did you go to bed?
8:30 p.m.

What was your favorite exercise?
i loved to box and spar in the gym

How many days a week did you train?
Six days

Did you have a job before you won the world title?
No

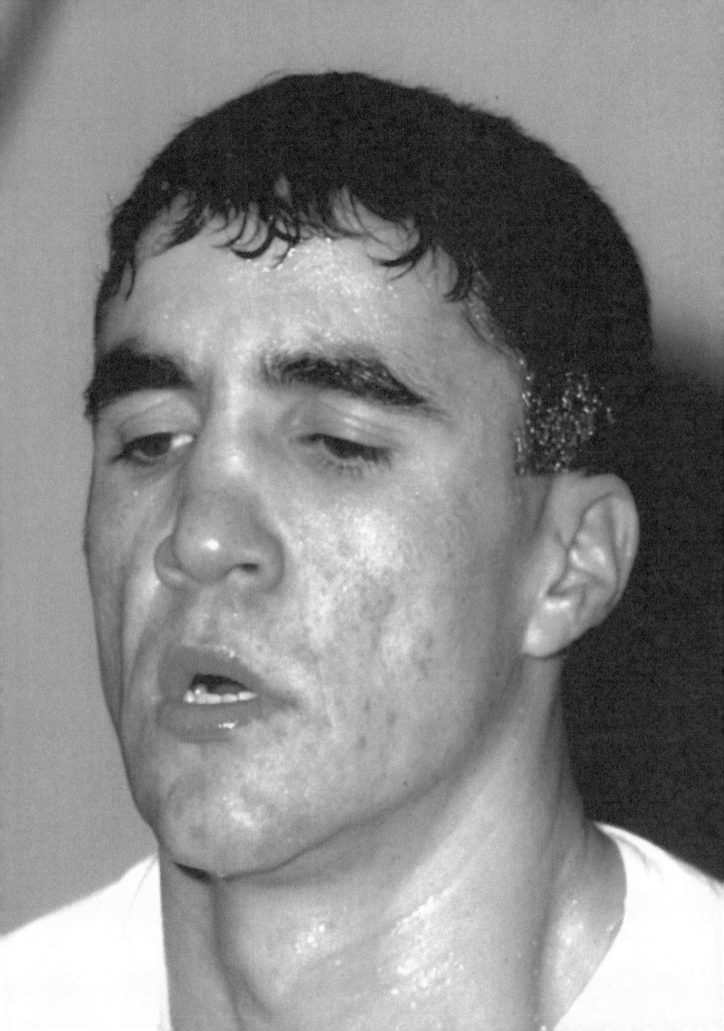

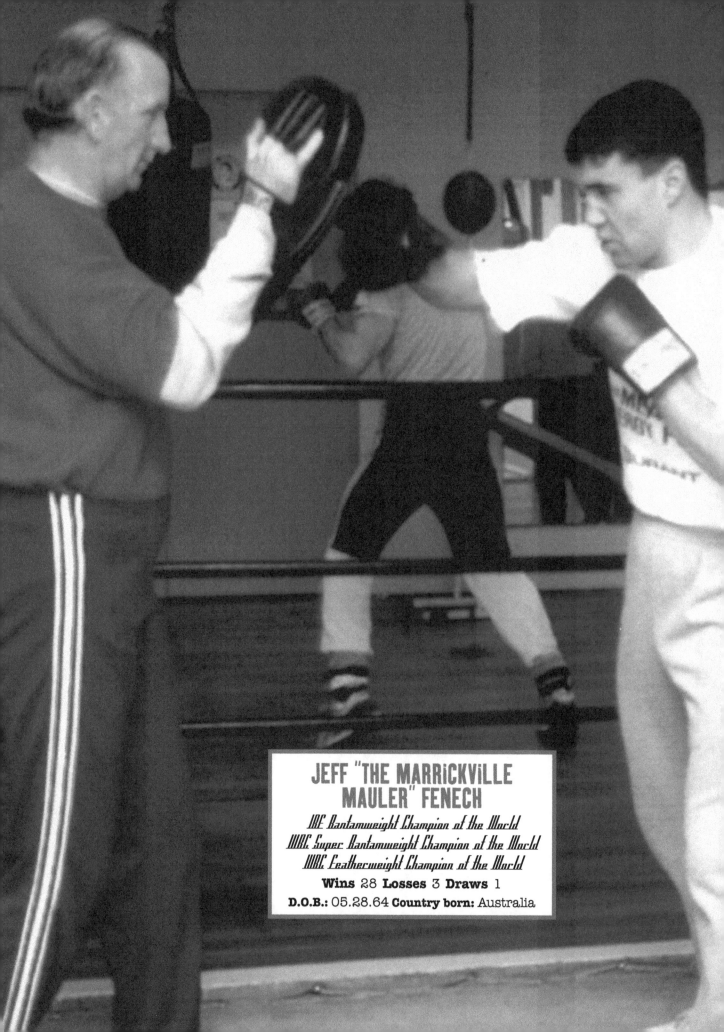

JEFF "THE MARRICKVILLE MAULER" FENECH

IBF Bantamweight Champion of the World
WBC Super Bantamweight Champion of the World
WBC Featherweight Champion of the World

Wins 28 **Losses** 3 **Draws** 1

D.O.B.: 05.28.64 **Country born:** Australia

JEFF FENECH'S
WORKOUT

SHADOWBOXING 4 x 3 minute rounds (30 second break after each round)

FOCUS PADS 6 x 3 minute rounds (30 second break after each round)

SPARRING in the weeks leading up to a fight, Jeff would cut down on the focus pads and add more sparring, building up the number of rounds: 3–12 x 3 minute rounds (30 second break between each round)

FLOOR-TO-CEILING BAG 9 minutes (followed by 30 second break)

JUMPING ROPE 12 minutes

FLOOR EXERCISES 5 x 20 push-ups (30 second break after each set)
15 x 20 sit-ups (30 second break after each set)
(Jeff always did 500 sit-ups over the day, each day)

JEFF HARDING

What time did you get up?
5:00 a.m.

Did you stretch before your run?
Yes, touched my toes and held, and did some side-to-sides and body swivels

How far did you run?
3–5 miles Monday, Wednesday, Friday and Sunday; 400-meter sprints with 1 minute break after each on Tuesday, Thursday and Saturday

What did you do after your run?
Had a shower and then breakfast

What did you eat for breakfast?
Porridge and banana, two pieces of toast with no butter, water

What did you do after breakfast?
Went for a walk, went to the shops and then met up with my promoter

What time did you go to the gym?
4:00 p.m.

What time did you leave the gym?
Around 6:00 p.m. (Monday to Friday)

What did you do after training?
Showered, then had my dinner

What did you eat for dinner?
A lot of carbos and steamed veggies, pasta, fish, chicken and fruit

What did you do after dinner?
i liked to play my guitar (i love the blues)

What time did you go to bed?
9:30 p.m.

What was your favorite exercise?
Focus pads

How many days a week did you train?
Seven days

Did you have a job before you won the world title?
Yes, i was a garbage collector with the local council

RING PRO
AUSTRALIA

JEFF "HiTMAN" HARDiNG
WBC Light Heavyweight Champion of the World
Wins 23 **Losses** 2 **Draws** 0
D.O.B.: 02.05.65 **Country born:** Australia

JEFF HARDING'S WORKOUT

WARM-UP	15 minutes in total body swivels (with or without a broom handle behind his neck) side-to-sides (with his hands reaching down to his knees) touching toes and holding for count of 10 bouncing around and swinging arms to get loose
SHADOWBOXING	3 x 3 minute rounds (30 second break after each round)
FOCUS PADS	3 x 3 minute rounds (30 second break after each round) 6 x 3 minute combinations (30 second break after each set)
FLOOR-TO-CEILING BAG	3 x 3 minute combinations (30 second break after each set)
JUMPING ROPE	9 minutes (followed by 30 second break)
FLOOR EXERCISES	5 x 20 push-ups 10 minutes of abdominal work
SPEED BAG	9 minutes
WARM-DOWN	15 minutes

KOSTYA TSZYU

What time do you get up?
7:00 a.m.

Do you stretch before your run?
Yes, always

How far do you run?
First i run up and down hills for 25 minutes,
then i do 30 minutes jogging on the road

What do you eat for breakfast?
Cereal, bran and milk

What do you do after breakfast?
Relax, sleep or conduct business

What time do you go to the gym?
2:00 p.m. i leave at 4:30–5:00 p.m.

What do you do after training?
Relax, go for a massage, then watch cable TV

What do you eat for dinner?
A lot of steamed vegetables (this is the key for me),
as well as chicken and fish. i also eat some red
meat, grilled.

What do you do after dinner?
Family is important to me, but i also like reading and
listening to Russian pop music

What time do you go to bed?
10:00 p.m.

What is your favorite exercise?
Anything that makes my body tired. i like everything,
but particularly weights.

How many days a week do you train?
Six days

Did you have a job before you won the world title?
Yes, i was in the Russian army

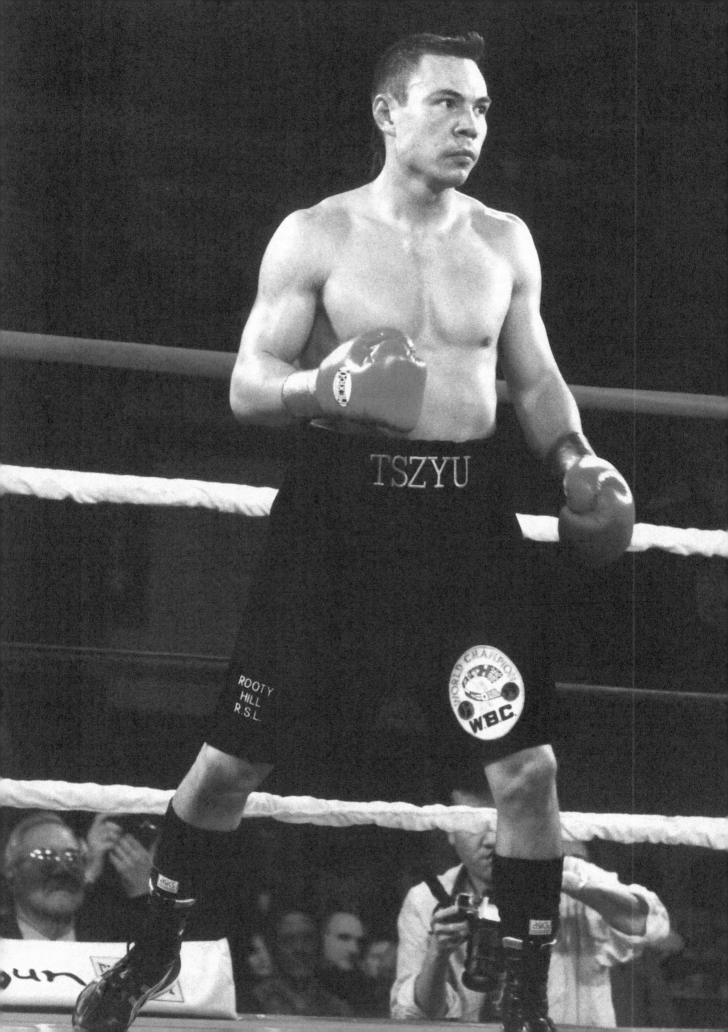

KOSTYA TSZYU'S WORKOUT

STRENGTH & INITIAL CONDITIONING WORKOUT

Kostya does this program to build up his strength before he moves on to the conventional boxing training (bag work, speed bag, focus pads and sparring).

WARM-UP	touch toes and hold for 10 seconds side-to-sides for 1 minute swing arms up and down, alternating for 1 minute bend knees and touch the floor with fingers
PUSH-UPS	50 on knuckles
PULL-UPS	10 using a close grip (followed by 30 second break)
JUMPING ROPE	20 minutes at moderate pace (followed by 1 minute break)
PULL-UPS	4 x 10 (30 second break after each set)
DUMBBELLS	4 x 1 minute rounds on alternating dumbbell curls (30 second break after each round then 1 minute break at end)
BARBELLS	4 x 15 barbell curls (30 second break after each set then 1 minute break at end)
BARBELL DISC	3 x 20 lifts (30 second break after each set) Pull disc up to your chest with both hands and let it fall back to your thighs.
BENCH PRESS	70 reps at 75 lbs.
NECK TWISTS & ROTATIONS	Lie flat on your back, lift your head up off the ground and move it up and down then around for 1 minute.
LEG-RAISES	1 minute (followed by 30 second break) Lie on your back, stretch out your legs, lift them off the floor and hold.

LEG-RAISES	4 x 1 minute holds (30 second break after each lift) As before, but lift legs all the way.
SIT-UPS	3 x 50 on floor (30 second break after each set)
	To finish walk around for 1 minute, then drink, then shower

BOXiNG WORKOUT

WARM-UP	Same as strength and conditioning workout
PUSH-UPS	50 on knuckles
JUMPiNG ROPE	20 minutes
HEAVY BAG	10 minutes
SHADOWBOXiNG	3 x 3 minute rounds (30 second break after each round)
SPARRiNG	6–12 x 3 minute rounds (30 second break after each round) (Kostya builds up to 12 rounds with 3 different sparring partners. You can do bag work instead of sparring.)
FOCUS PADS	6 x 3 minute rounds working on combinations (30 second break after each round)
SHADOWBOXiNG	3 minute round at slow pace (followed by 30 second break)
GYMNASTiCS	standing on his head in the middle of the ring, balancing and focusing (about 3 minutes), then tumbling around the ring without stopping for approximately 25 revolutions
SPEED BAG	3 minutes (30 second break)
TENNiS BALL	Kostya has his own way of fine-tuning his hand–eye coordination. He uses a band around his head, which has a length of elastic attached to it (see opposite). Attached to the other end of the elastic is a tennis ball that he punches out with his fists. He aims to get into a steady rhythm, keeping the tennis ball and his fists moving until his chosen time is up on the clock.
JUMPiNG ROPE	10 minutes
TO FiNiSH	rub down, drink and shower

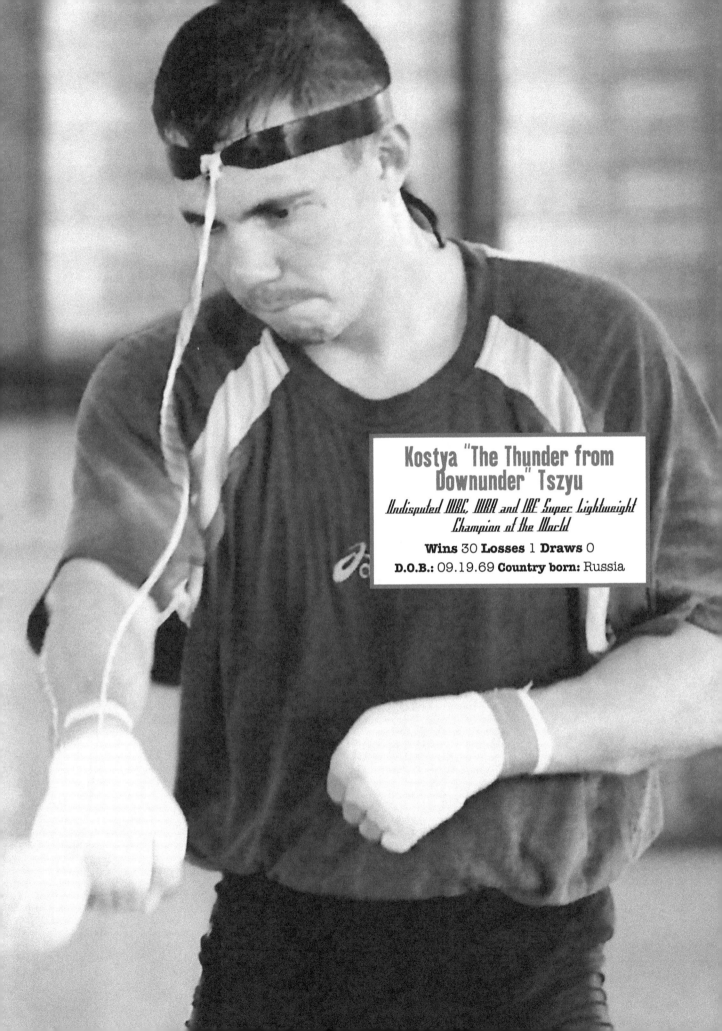

Kostya "The Thunder from Downunder" Tszyu

Undisputed WBC, WBA and IBF Super Lightweight Champion of the World

Wins 30 **Losses** 1 **Draws** 0

D.O.B.: 09.19.69 **Country born:** Russia

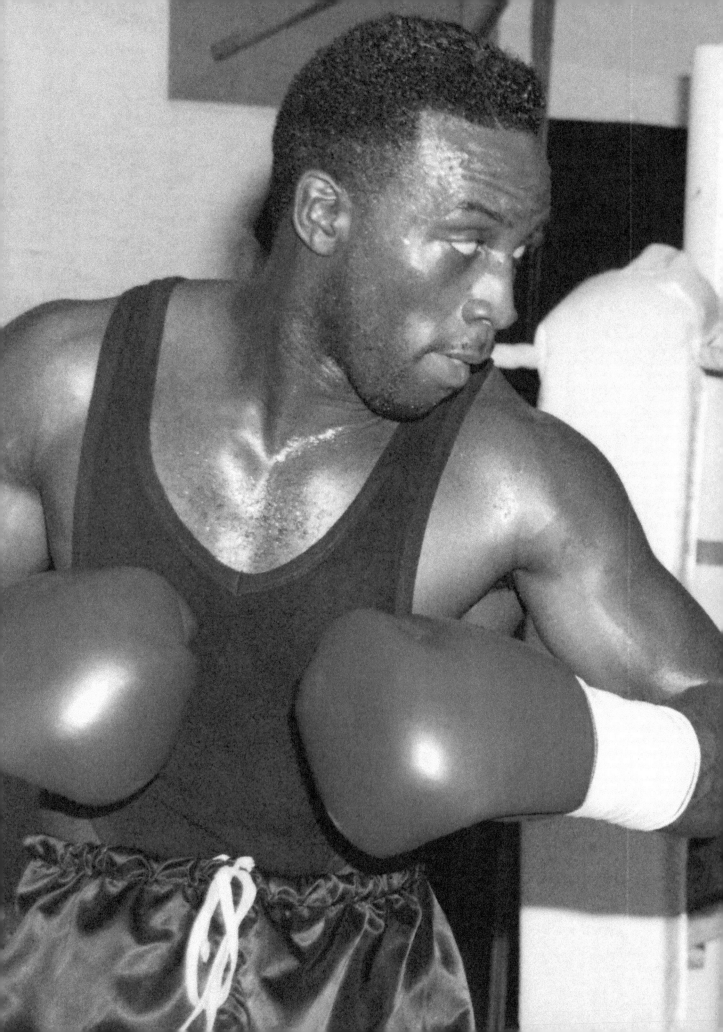

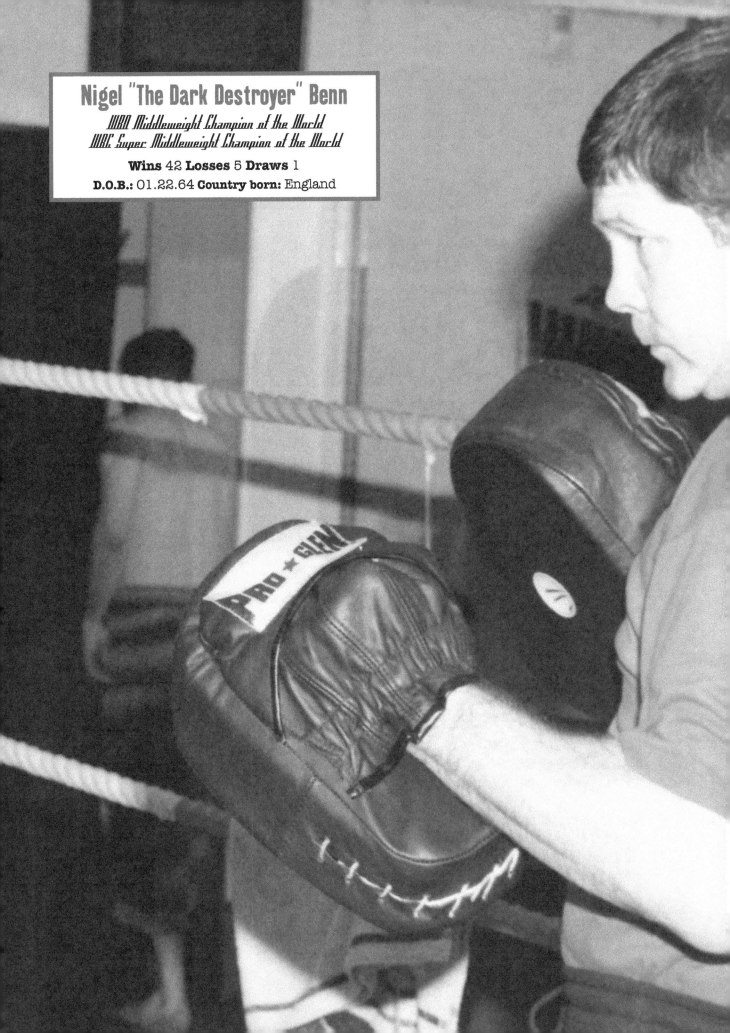

Nigel "The Dark Destroyer" Benn

WBO Middleweight Champion of the World
WBC Super Middleweight Champion of the World

Wins 42 **Losses** 5 **Draws** 1

D.O.B.: 01.22.64 **Country born:** England

NiGEL BENN

What time do you get up?
7:00 a.m. i have breakfast, then i have to travel to my running site up in the mountains.

Do you stretch before your run?
Yes, full stretch

How far do you run?
i run at altitude. i start off at 6–8 miles and build up to 12–15 miles at my peak. i cut down on the miles about 4 weeks before i fight.

What do you do after your run?
Travel back to home base and get ready for my first workout session

What do you eat for breakfast?
Porridge and banana, and i also have my vitamin tablets with vegetable juices and water

What do you do to get ready for your run?
Get my gear ready (Walkman, ankle weights, etc.), then travel to the site, which is nearly one hour away

What time do you go to the gym?
About 11:30 a.m. for my first session, then i rest and prepare for the next training session

What time do you leave the gym?
Around 7:00 p.m.

What do you do after training?
Shower, and have dinner

What do you eat for dinner?
i like turkey, chicken, vegetables, salmon, sweet potatoes (no butter or salt) and pasta. i also have more multivitamins and an iron tablet (with zinc, potassium and calcium).

What do you do after dinner?
To relax, i like to play my PlayStation or listen to music. Sometimes i do a bit of DJ-ing at a club.

What time do you go to bed?
it depends on how i feel

What is your favorite exercise?
Focus pads, and i love going out running in the mountains

How many days a week do you train?
i train every day, but sometimes i take off and chill out. i always come back stronger.

Did you have a job before you won the world title?
Yes, i was in the army. it's also where i started to box.

NiGEL BENN'S WORKOUT

WARM-UP	touching toes and holding side-to-sides rotating hips swiveling torso while holding a long stick behind neck swinging arms back and forth at sides, and in and out from sides
SHADOWBOXiNG	3 x 3 rounds with 15-pound hand weights (30 second break after each round) 2 x 3 minute rounds without hand weights (30 second break after each round)
FOCUS PADS	4 x 3 minute rounds working on stamina and combinations (30 second break after each round)
FLOOR-TO-CEiLiNG BAG	3 x 3 minute rounds (30 second break after each round)
JUMPiNG ROPE	20 minutes (followed by 1 minute break)
FLOOR EXERCISES	4 x 25 sit-ups Do this with a partner pushing you down fast as you sit up—very fast and explosive. 4 x 25 leg-raises 4 x 25 stand-up/sit-ups 4 x 25 cross-overs Lie on your back and stretch out your legs. Lift your feet off the floor and cross them over each other, alternating which foot is on top. 4 x 25 push-ups Do these with your hands as far apart as you can manage.

TO FiNiSH   walk around for 1 minute

Nigel did his usual workout every day, but added a weight program every second day, working every muscle, including his neck. He used a harness on his head from which he suspended weights fitted to a strap. He would also get a partner to pull down on the strap for a period of time while he took the strain. Nigel didn't spar that much — he saved it for the fight.

stand-up/sit-ups

This really tests your stomach and legs. Lie down on your back with a partner positioned at your feet. Sit up as if you are going to do a normal sit-up. At this point, your partner takes the backs of your knees, and while you push off with your legs and stomach, your partner helps you up. Once you are up, stand straight for a second and then repeat. Continue at a fast pace.

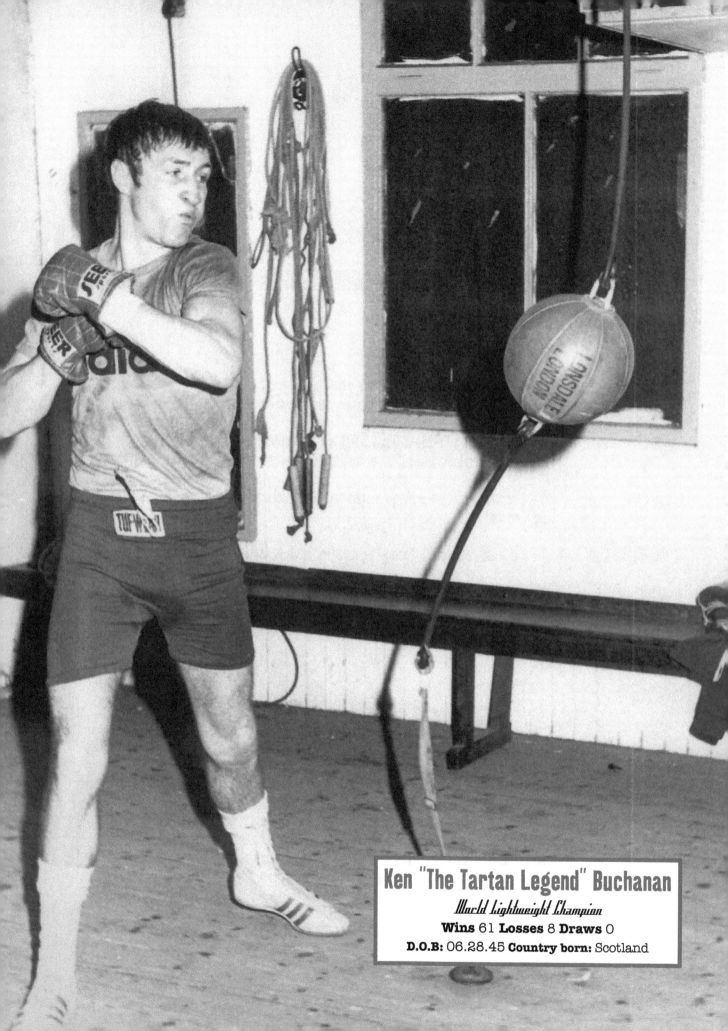

Ken "The Tartan Legend" Buchanan
World Lightweight Champion
Wins 61 **Losses** 8 **Draws** 0
D.O.B: 06.28.45 **Country born:** Scotland

KEN BUCHANAN

What time did you get up?
6:00 a.m.

Did you stretch before your run?
Yes, full warm-up and a good stretch

How far did you run?
i usually ran for about 6 miles or 1 hour, and i always fitted in short bursts of sprints along the way. All through my career i ran with heavy army-type boots on. All the "old school" did this.

What did you do after your run?
i had a bath and then i went to bed until about 11:30 a.m.

What did you eat for breakfast?
i liked scrambled eggs, bacon and toast with honey. i also had cod liver oil tablets to help lubricate the muscles, and also salt tablets before breakfast.

What did you do after breakfast?
i liked to watch films or i would go swimming. i also enjoyed the odd game of golf and listening to Neil Diamond records.

What time did you eat dinner?
4:00 p.m.

What did you eat for dinner?
Always high protein, chicken or steak with vegetables

What time did you go to the gym?
6:30 p.m. i'd leave at 8:30–9.00 p.m.

What did you do after training?
Had a bath, watched TV

What time did you go to bed?
Around 10:30 p.m. with a cup of hot chocolate

What was your favorite exercise?
Sparring. And i loved swimming. i'd swim underwater as long as i could until i thought my lungs would burst. Great way to expand the lungs.

How many days a week did you train?
Five days

Did you have a job before you won the world title?
Yes, i was a joiner (carpenter)

KEN BUCHANAN'S WORKOUT

WARM-UP	stretching for 20 minutes: side-to-sides touching toes and holding swinging arms up and down swiveling torso jumping about on toes (going straight into shadowboxing)
SHADOWBOXING	3 x 3 minute rounds (30 second break after each round)
SPARRING	8 x 3 minute rounds (30 second break after each round) (Ken split up the sparring with heavy bag work: 4 x 3 minutes on the heavy bag with 30 second break; 4 x 3 minutes sparring with 30 second break)
JUMPING ROPE	30 minutes (followed by 1 minute break)
FLOOR EXERCISES	push-ups sit-ups leg-raises lots of abdominal work with the medicine ball light weights exercises (25 minutes in total)
WEIGHTS	light weights with high repetitions

Strength-building

Lie on the floor on your back. Stretch out your arms all the way behind your head and shoulders. Lift the barbell and hold 6 inches off the ground. Hold until you reach your maximum, then lower to the floor. Rest for 15 seconds, then repeat until you reach your max.

TO FINISH Ken would wrap himself (including his head) in a big towel and sweat out until his temperature stabilized. Then he had a drink, and went home for a bath and to relax

WAYNE McCULLOUGH

What time do you get up?
I love to run in the desert. As it's so hot in Las Vegas, i run at around 8 a.m. in the winter months i run at around 9 a.m.

Do you stretch before you run?
Only light stretching, because i tend to pull my muscles

How far do you run?
5 miles a day, 6 days a week

After running, what do you do?
Shadowboxing and then sit-ups, and push-ups before cooling down

What do you eat for breakfast?
Fruit juice, yogurt, fruit and toast

What time do you go to the gym?
I go to the gym at around 4 p.m. and finish at around 6 p.m. if i am sparring, i will be a little longer

What do you do after training?
I relax and wind down from the adrenaline rush of being in the ring

What do you have for dinner?
Chicken with pasta, potatoes or rice on the side.

Do you have any hobbies?
I love playing golf and riding my Harley Davidson motorbike around Las Vegas. i also enjoy taking my little girl bowling or to the movies.

What do you do after dinner?
Watch a DVD or go to the movies

What time do you go to bed?
When i'm in training for a fight, i go to bed at 10 p.m. so i can get up early to run

What is your favorite exercise?
Sit-ups on an exercise ball. i hold a 20-pound plate behind my head while balancing on the ball, and continue to do sit-ups.

How many days do you train?
Seven days a week, with a light workout on Sunday. i have always done this throughout my career. When Eddie Futch trained me, he couldn't get me to take a day off training.

Did you have a job before you won the world title?
I started boxing at the age of 8 and i didn't turn pro until i was 22. When i left school, i worked on a training scheme where i studied carpentry, which i loved. i then worked as a care-taker in a church in Belfast. After that, i went to the Olympics—and the rest is history.

WAYNE McCULLOUGH'S WORKOUT

WARM-UP	10 minutes, non-stop (30 second break)
SHADOWBOXING	6 x 3 minute rounds (30 second break)
SPARRING	4–8 rounds x 3 minute rounds on sparring days (60 second break after each 3 mins)
FOCUS PADS	2 x 3 minute rounds 5 x 3 minute rounds on non-sparring days
FLOOR-TO-CEILING BAG	2 x 3 minute rounds (30 second break)
SPEED BAG	2 x 3 minute rounds (30 second break)
HEAVY BAG	4 x 3 minute rounds (on days when not sparring)
JUMPING ROPE	10 minutes non-stop (30 second break)
FLOOR WORK	sit-ups (200 total) push-ups (150 total) pull-ups (2 sets of 15 repetitions) bar dips (2 x sets of 40 repetitions)
LIGHT WEIGHTS	light barbells or dumbbells with maximum repetitions
WARM-DOWN	light stretching to all the muscles
TO FINISH	shower and relax

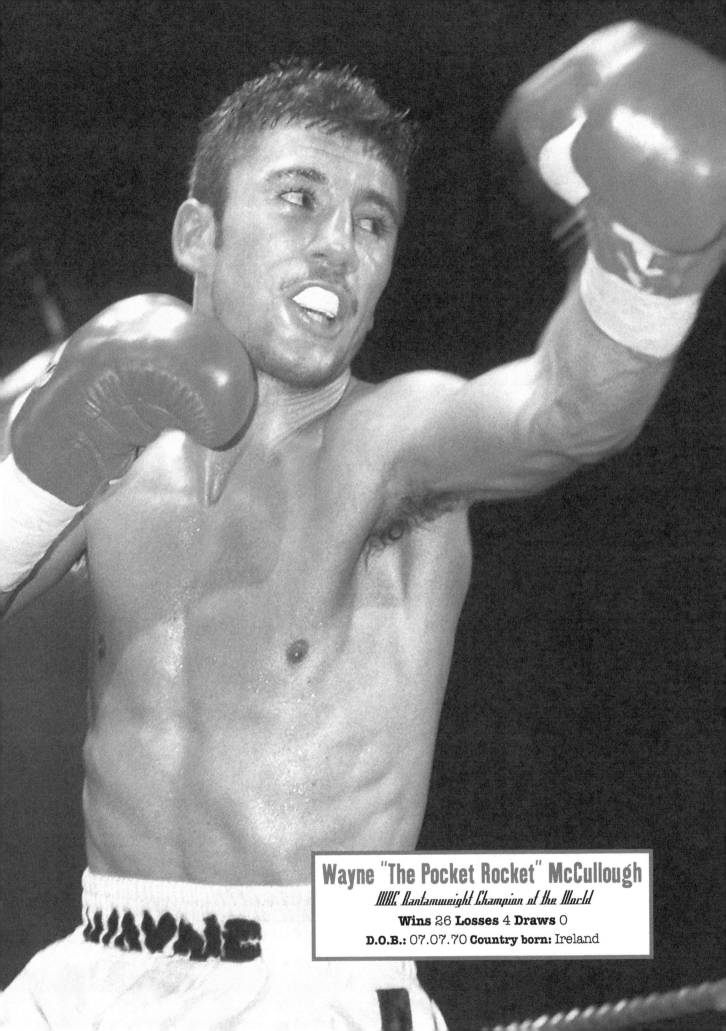

Wayne "The Pocket Rocket" McCullough
WBC Bantamweight Champion of the World
Wins 26 **Losses** 4 **Draws** 0
D.O.B.: 07.07.70 **Country born:** Ireland

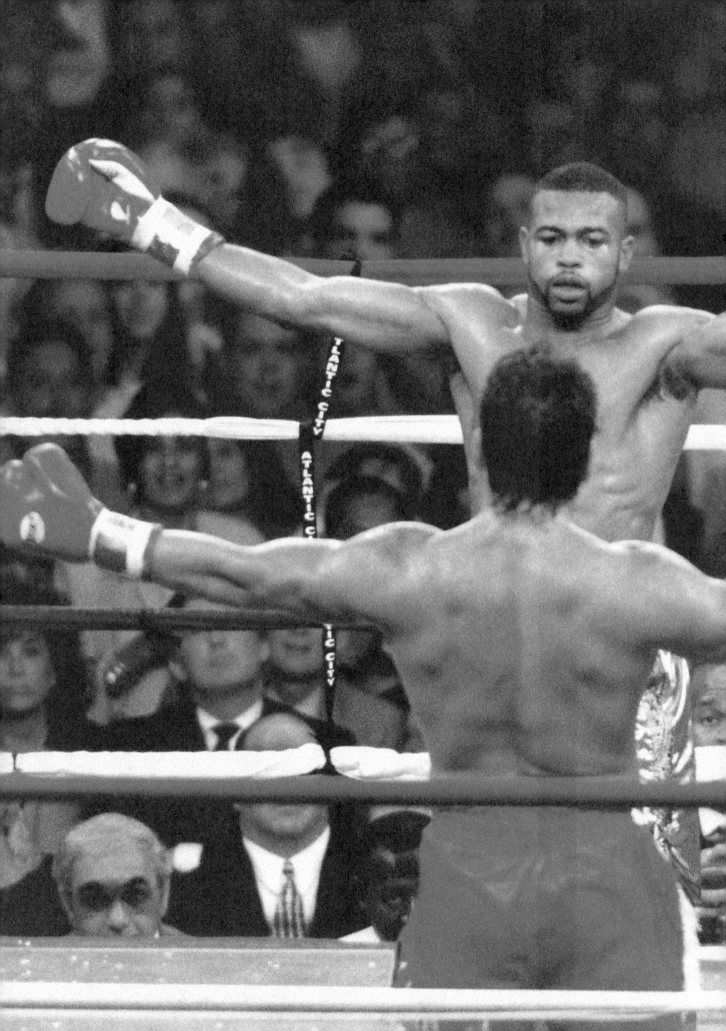

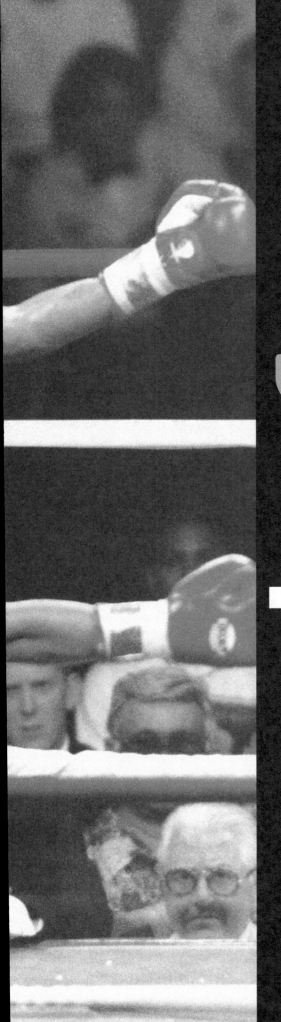

ROY JONES JUNIOR

What time do you get up?
5:30 a.m.

Do you stretch before your run?
Yes, i do a full body warm-up. i stretch my
legs, back, sides and mid-section.

How far do you run?
Around 3–5 miles

What do you do after your run?
i always do leg weights, light with lots of reps.
i then have a shower and rest.

What do you eat for breakfast?
i like scrambled eggs and hash browns, then fruit

What do you do after breakfast?
Sleep

What time do you go to the gym?
12:00 midday

What time do you leave the gym?
3:30 p.m.

What do you do after training?
Play basketball

What do you eat for dinner?
i like turkey, chicken, pasta and plenty of vegetables.
i always eat nutritious food.

What do you do after dinner?
i love to play with my kids and hang out. It helps me
relax. i also like to play on the computer.

What time do you go to bed?
10:30 p.m.

What is your favorite exercise?
i love to work out, but i would have to say stomach
exercises

How many days a week do you train?
Five or six days

Did you have a job before you won the world title?
No

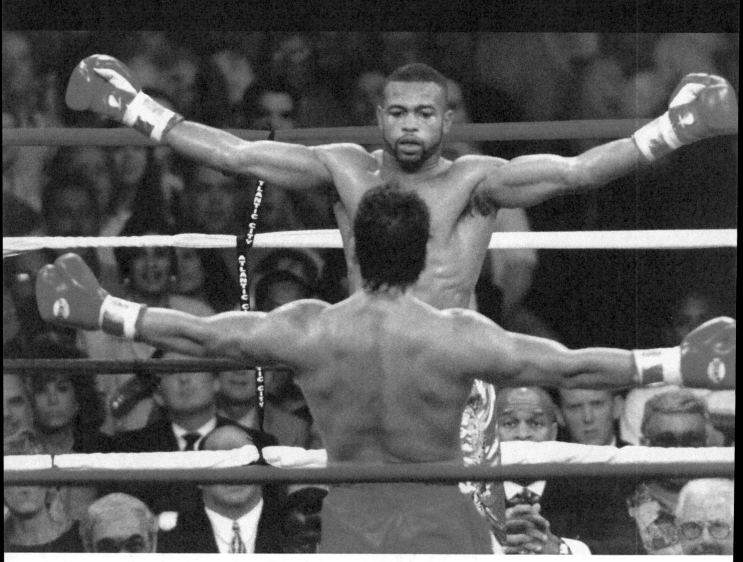

WORKOUTS FROM BOXING'S GREATEST CHAMPS

ROY JONES, JR.'S WORKOUT

WARM-UP	touching toes and holding side-to-sides torso twists push-ups full body stretch bouncing around on toes while moving around
SHADOWBOXING	4 x 4 minute rounds (30 second break after each round)
HEAVY BAG	4 x 4 minute rounds (30 second break after each round)
SPEED BAG	16 minutes (followed by 30 second break)
FLOOR-TO-CEILING BAG	16 minutes (followed by 30 second break)
JUMPING ROPE	25 minutes at steady pace (followed by 1 minute break)
ABDOMINAL WORK	4 x 100 sit-ups (30 second break after each set) 4 x 100 leg-raises (30 second break after each set) 4 x 100 crunches (30 second break after each set)

Roy does not use weights in his workout

Roy Jones, Junior

IBF Middleweight Champion of the World
IBF Super Middleweight Champion of the World
WBA, WBC, IBF and IBO Light Heavyweight Champion of the World
WBA Heavyweight Champion of the World
WBC, IBO Light Heavyweight Champion of the World

Wins 49 **Losses** 1 **Draws** 0
D.O.B.: 01.16.69 **Country born:** U.S.A.

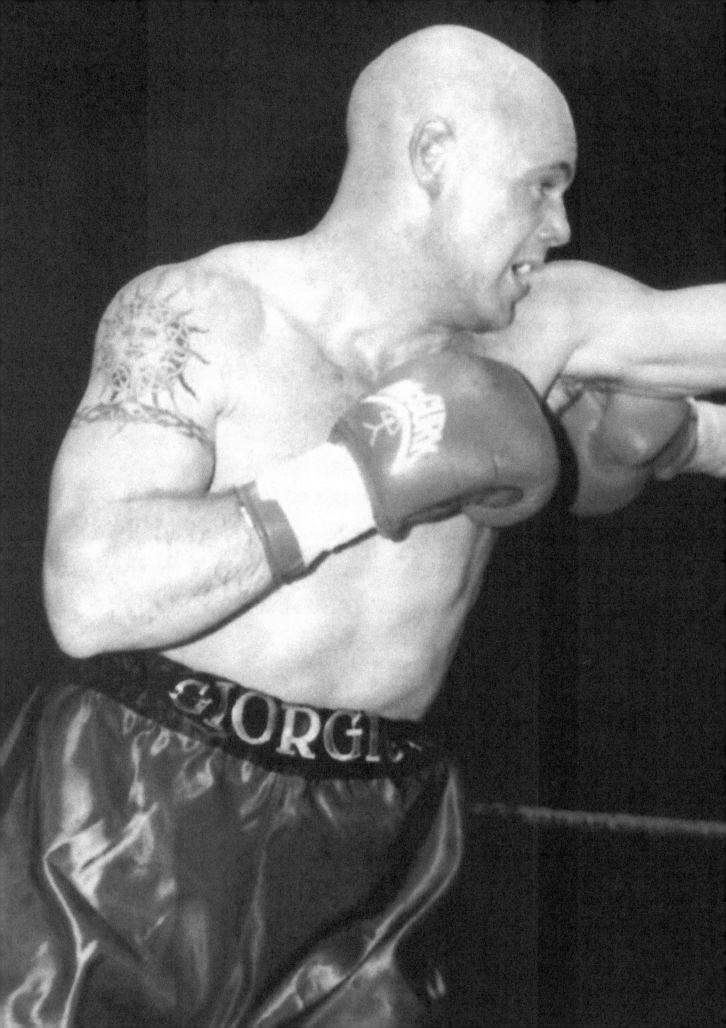

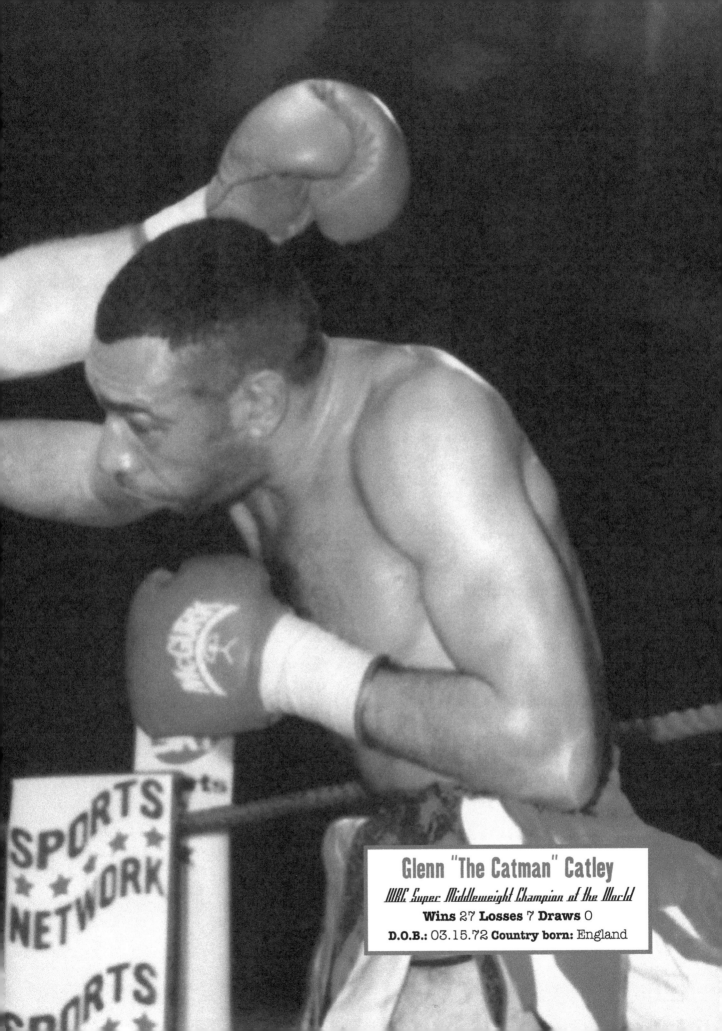

Glenn "The Catman" Catley
WBC Super Middleweight Champion of the World
Wins 27 **Losses** 7 **Draws** 0
D.O.B.: 03.15.72 **Country born:** England

GLENN CATLEY

What time do you get up?
7:00 a.m. i don't run in the morning because it suits me better to run at 5:00 p.m.

What do you eat for breakfast?
Cereal and milk, two boiled eggs and bread

What do you do after breakfast?
i take my kids to school around 9:00 a.m.

What time do you go to the gym?
10:00 a.m.

What time do you leave the gym?
1:00 p.m.

What do you do after training?
i usually stay at the gym, have some fruit and watch videos of the guy i will be fighting. On Monday, Wednesday and Friday, i go with my strength conditioner, and we do 1 hour of strength exercises.

How far do you run?
i'm out on the road for about 40 minutes, and it adds up to around 5 miles

Do you stretch before your run?
No

What do you eat for dinner?
i like fish, broccoli, carrots and i love cabbage. i eat a lot of vegetables.

What do you do after dinner?
i play with my kids, then get their pajamas on for bed. Then i have a relaxing evening with my wife.

What time do you go to bed?
10:00 p.m.

What is your favorite exercise?
Focus pads

How many days a week do you train?
Six days, with Sunday off

Did you have a job before you won the world title?
Yes, i worked as an electrician

GLENN CATLEY'S
WORKOUT

WARM-UP — dancing around on toes for approximately 20 minutes

FOCUS PADS — 6–14 x 3 minute rounds (30 second break after each round), building up as his training camp progresses, working on technique, combinations and hooks

HEAVY BAG — 6 x 1 minute rounds (1 minute break after each round)
Glenn always does this with a partner. They take turns punching hard and fast for 1 minute, while the other holds the bag. The partner counts up to 20 and down to 1 as the other punches.

SPEED BAG — 5 minutes (followed by 30 second break)

JUMPING ROPE — 20 minutes (followed by 1 minute break)

CIRCUIT ON FLOOR — repeat all exercises as many times as you can in 20 minutes:

1 bench press (50 lb. maximum weight) for 30 seconds only
2 sit-ups for 30 seconds only
3 trampoline jumps (raising knees) for 30 seconds only
4 push-ups for 30 seconds only
5 stepping up and down off a 500 mm bench for 30 seconds only
6 lifting light weights above head for 30 seconds only
7 jumping jacks for 30 seconds only
8 squat thrusts for 30 seconds only

Squat Thrusts
Crouch down with hands on the floor in front of you. Throw both feet out behind you, straightening your legs. Bring both legs up into a crouching position so that your knees hit your elbows. Then go straight back into starting position. This should be continuous and explosive.

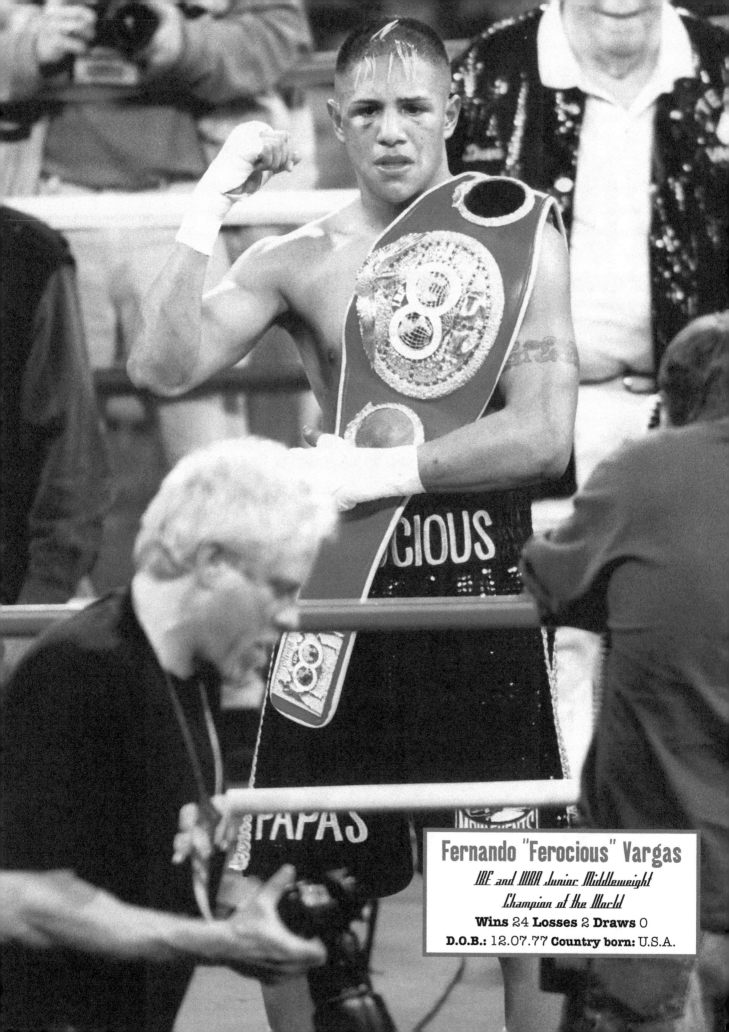

Fernando "Ferocious" Vargas
IBF and WBA Junior Middleweight
Champion of the World
Wins 24 **Losses** 2 **Draws** 0
D.O.B.: 12.07.77 **Country born:** U.S.A.

FERNANDO VARGAS

What time do you get up?
7:00 a.m.

Do you stretch before your run?
Yes, full stretch to the legs and back

How far do you run?
4–7 miles

What do you do after your run?
i stretch down and have a shower before breakfast

What do you eat for breakfast?
Fruit, fruit juice and i also drink water. i also like eggs, hash browns and pancakes in between fights.

What do you do after breakfast?
i rest and then get focused on my workout

What time do you go to the gym?
9:00 a.m.

What time do you leave the gym?
11:30 a.m.

What do you do after training?
Sometimes i get a rub-down, have a shower, then do some promo work. i also like to do charity work for the little kids.

What do you eat for dinner?
i like chicken, rice and salad

What do you do after dinner?
Watch TV, and i like to play pool with my Team Vargas family. My family is very important to me. i also like to listen to music and hang out.

What time do you go to bed?
Around 10:00 p.m.

What is your favorite exercise?
i love training hard. i enjoy it all.

How many days a week do you train?
Six days

Did you have a job before you won the world title?
No

FERNANDO VARGAS WORKOUT

WARM-UP	15 minutes of full body stretch and warm-up
SHADOWBOXiNG	3 x 3 minute rounds (30 second break after each round)
FOCUS PADS	6 x 3 minute rounds (30 second break after each round)
HEAVY BAG	6 x 3 minute rounds (30 second break after each round) (if sparring, cut back on the focus pads and the heavy bag)
FLOOR-TO-CEILiNG BAG	5 minutes (followed by 30 second break)
SPEED BAG	5 minutes (followed by 30 second break)
FLOOR EXERCiSES	abdominal exercises sit-ups 8 x 50 leg-raises (various types) 3 x 20 dips on the bars 3 x 20 pull-ups resistance training with thera-bands (elastic resistance bands)
JUMPiNG ROPE	20 minutes
WARM-DOWN	5 minutes of stretching, then walk around
TO FiNiSH	rub-down

KEN
NORTON

did you get up?

retch before your run?
ody stretch

d you run?
from 3–8 miles, depending on my progress
camp

ou do after your run?
n for 15 minutes, then i would take a
hen i'd eat

ou eat for breakfast?
ve nine eggs, seven pieces of bacon, eight
toast, a bowl of cereal, two glasses of
ce and two glasses of milk

ou do after breakfast?
a walk for 3 miles, then i came home

did you go to the gym?

What time did you leave the gym?
3:30 p.m.

What did you do after training?
Rested my body and relaxed

What did you eat for dinner?
i had my meal around 5:30 p.m. i would have two big
steaks, some beans and lots of vegetables.

What did you do after dinner?
i liked to watch movies, and also fight tapes of the
individual i was going to be fighting

What time did you go to bed?
10:30 p.m.

What was your favorite exercise?
Everything

How many days a week did you train?
Six, with Sunday off

Did you have a job before you won the world title?
Yes, i was in the Marines for four-and-a-half years

KEN NORTON'S WORKOUT

WARM-UP	20 minutes of full body stretching
SHADOWBOXiNG	3 x 3 minute rounds (30 second break after each round)
SPARRiNG	3–9 x 3 minute rounds (30 second break after each round) with three sparring partners, depending on progress in training camp
HEAVY BAG	3 x 3 minute rounds (30 second break after each round)
SPEED BAG	3 x 3 minute rounds (30 second break after each round)
FLOOR-TO-CEiLiNG BAG	3 x 3 minute rounds (30 second break after each round)
SHADOWBOXiNG	3 x 3 minute rounds (30 second break after each round)
FLOOR EXERCiSES	250–300 sit-ups 250 leg-raises stretching (30 minutes in total)
TO FiNiSH	shower and rest

KEN "HERCULES" NORTON
WBC Heavyweight Champion of the World
Wins 42 **Losses** 7 **Draws** 1
D.O.B.: 09.08.43 **Country born:** U.S.A.

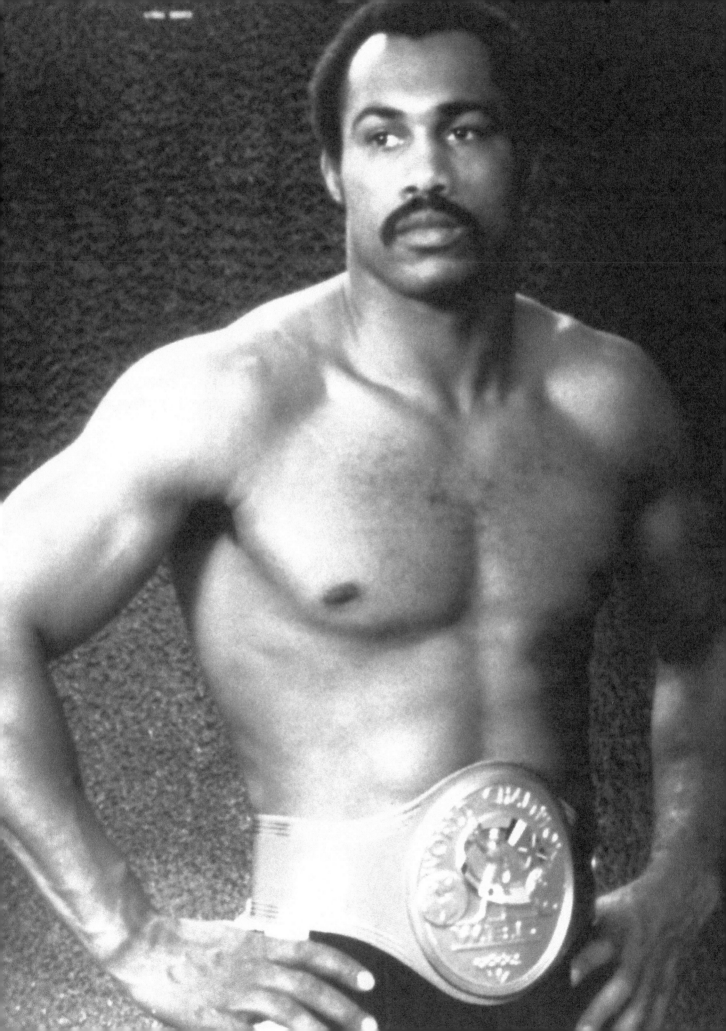

MUHAMMAD ALi

What time did you get up?
Very early, around 5:30 a.m. to run

Did you stretch before your run?
Yes, light stretching

How far did you run?
i ran about 6 miles, which took about 40 minutes
(i always ran in army-type boots)

What did you do after your run?
i did some exercises, stretching, and back home to
get washed up

What did you eat for breakfast?
All natural foods, orange juice and water

What did you do after breakfast?
i was always busy with public engagements and
newspaper people. i loved to meet the people.

What time did you go to the gym?
12:30 p.m.

What time did you leave the gym?
3:30 p.m.

What did you do after training?
i had a rub-down, then washed up. i would maybe talk
with the TV people, go out and enjoy myself, then eat.

What did you eat for dinner?
i always ate good: chicken, steaks, green beans,
potatoes, vegetables, fruit, juice and water

What did you do after dinner?
i liked to go for a walk, and watch TV

What time did you go to bed?
That depended on how i was feeling

What was your favorite exercise?
Shadowboxing and jumping rope. i loved gymwork.

How many days a week did you train?
Six days

Did you have a job before you won the world title?
No

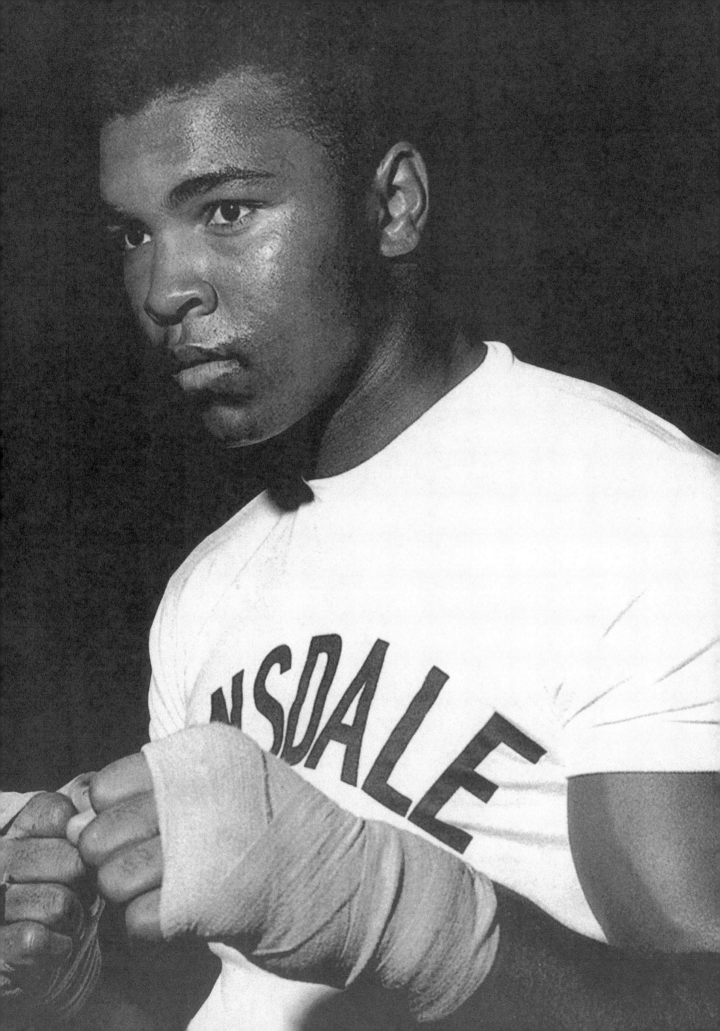

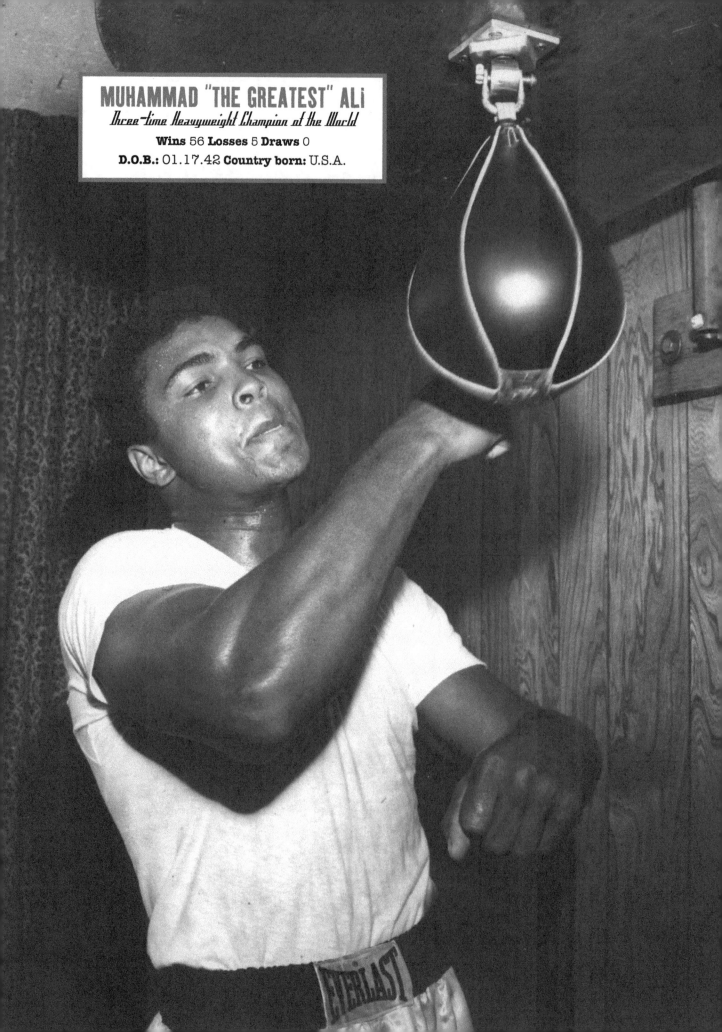

MUHAMMAD "THE GREATEST" ALi
Three-time Heavyweight Champion of the World
Wins 56 **Losses** 5 **Draws** 0
D.O.B.: 01.17.42 **Country born:** U.S.A.

MUHAMMAD ALI'S WORKOUT

WARM-UP	**side-to-sides** **torso swivels** **jumping around on toes to limber up** **(15 minutes in total)**
SHADOWBOXiNG	**5 x 3 minute rounds, working on footwork and speed punching** **(30 second break after each round)**
HEAVY BAG	**6 x 3 minute rounds, working on combinations and stamina** **(30 second break after each round)**
SPARRiNG	**built up sparring as training camp progressed**
FLOOR EXERCiSES	**15 minutes of exercises (300 in total)** **sit-ups in bicycling motion** **sit-ups with a medicine ball** **leg-raises**
SPEED BAG	**9 minutes (followed by 1 minute break)**
JUMPiNG ROPE	**20 minutes (Ali always moved around: forward, backward and mixing it up, never staying in the same spot)**
SHADOWBOXiNG	**1 minute, walking around with light shadowboxing**
	Ali did not use weights in his workout

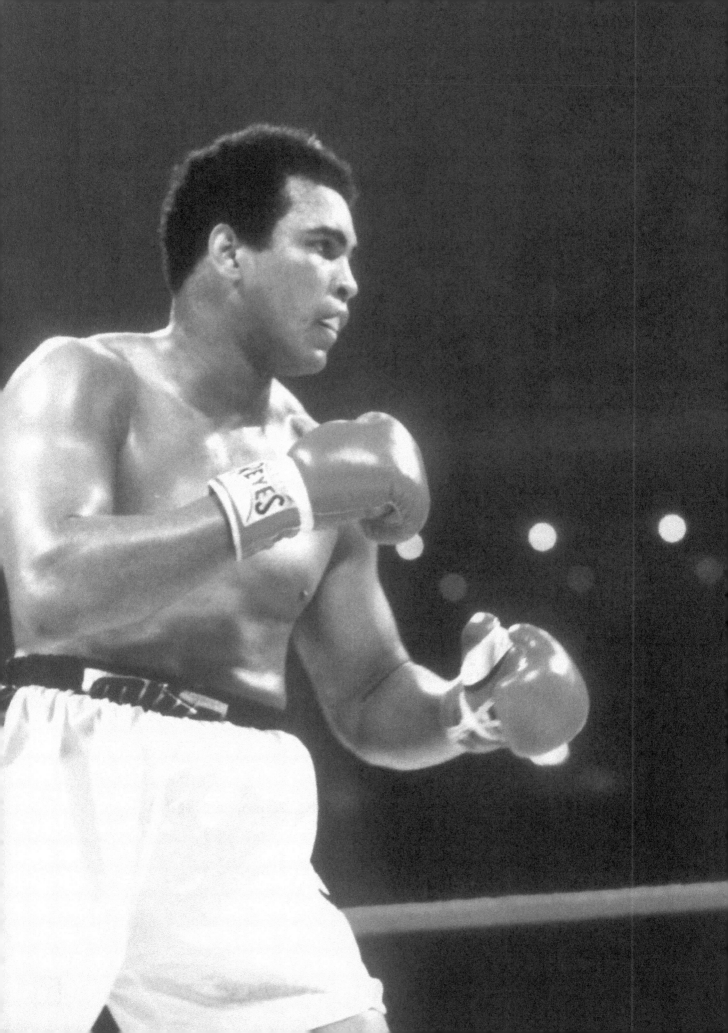

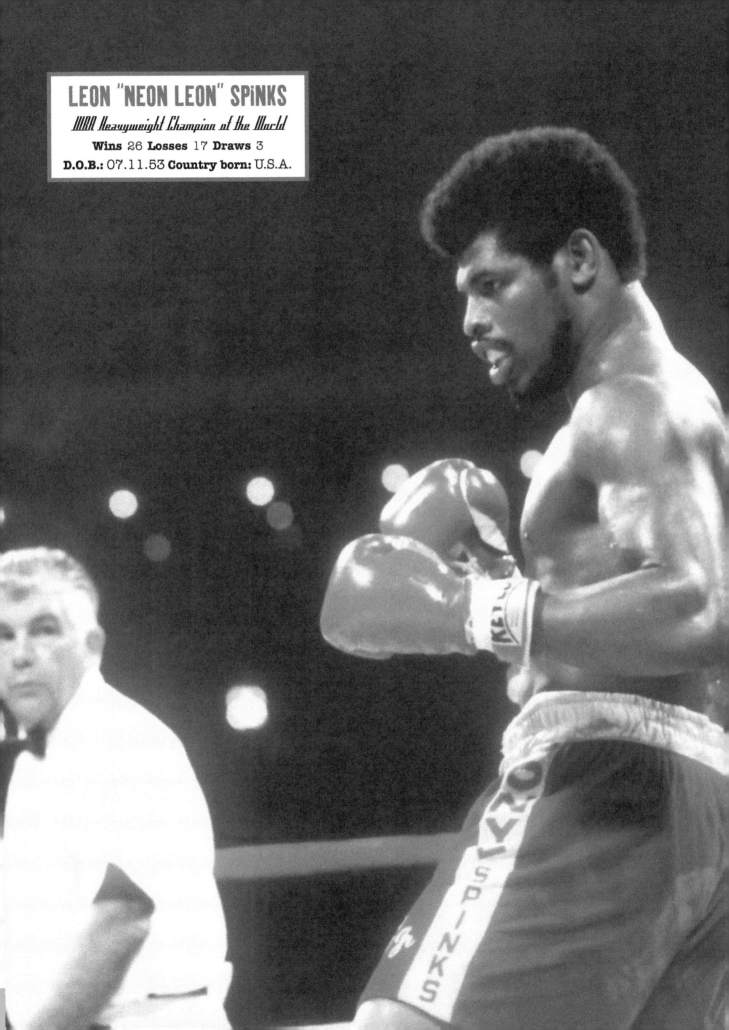

LEON "NEON LEON" SPINKS

WBA Heavyweight Champion of the World

Wins 26 **Losses** 17 **Draws** 3

D.O.B.: 07.11.53 **Country born:** U.S.A.

LEON SPINKS

What time did you get up?
6:00 a.m.

Did you stretch before your run?
Yes, full body stretch

How far did you run?
6 miles a day (Sunday off)

What did you do after your run?
i had some breakfast, then i went to sleep

What did you eat for breakfast?
Four eggs (soft), toast and fruit juice

What time did you go to the gym?
1:00 p.m. and i stayed there all day

What time did you leave the gym?
6:00 p.m. i used to hang out there and talk to the kids and help out where i could.

What did you do after training?
Talked to the kids in the neighborhood and maybe watched some TV

What did you eat for dinner?
i liked steak and a lot of vegetables

What did you do after dinner?
i watched some TV, then i set off for bed around 10:00 p.m.

What was your favorite exercise?
i liked to jump rope

How many days a week did you train?
Six days, with Sunday off

Did you have a job before you won the world title?
No

LEON SPINKS'S WORKOUT

WARM-UP	side-to-sides torso twists alternate arm swings leg-stretching, holding for 10 seconds
SPARRING	4 x 3 minute rounds (30 second break after each round) (Depending on his progress in training camp, Leon would mix sparring up with heavy bag work)
HEAVY BAG	5–8 x 3 minute rounds (30 second break after each round)
JUMPING ROPE	20 minutes (followed by 1 minute break walking around)
FLOOR EXERCISES	20 minutes in total: sit-ups leg-raises push-ups stretching out
TO FINISH	keep warm and rest

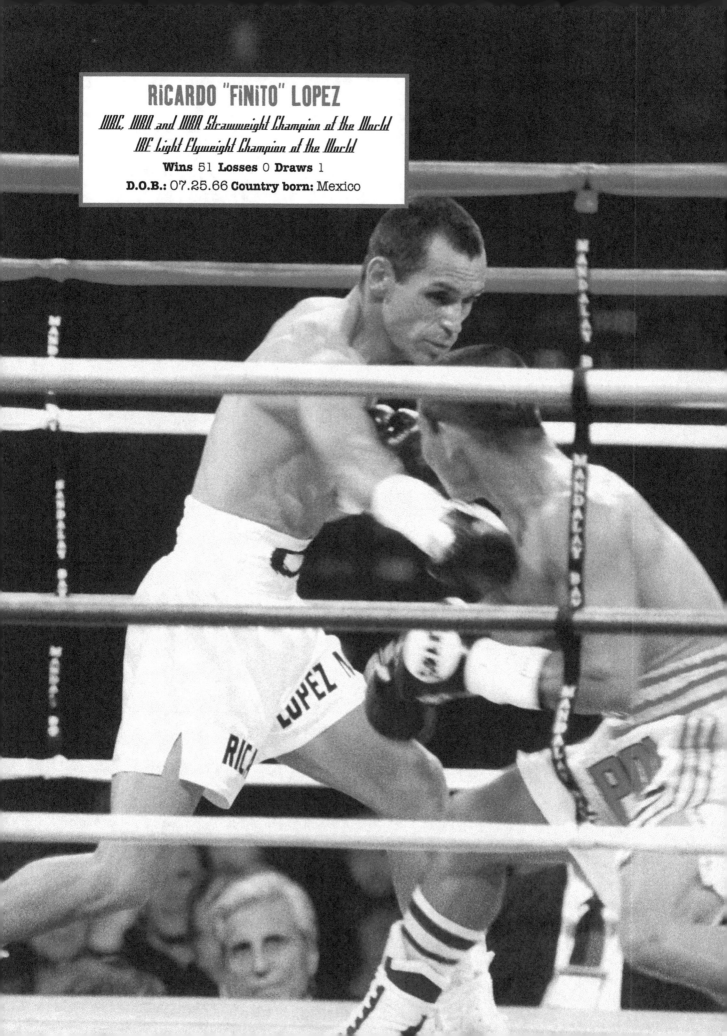

RiCARDO "FiNiTO" LOPEZ

WBC, WBO and WBA Strawweight Champion of the World
IBF Light Flyweight Champion of the World

Wins 51 **Losses** 0 **Draws** 1
D.O.B.: 07.25.66 **Country born:** Mexico

RICARDO LOPEZ

What time did you get up?
4:45 a.m.

Did you stretch before your run?
Yes, a good body stretch

How far did you run?
6–9 miles a day

What did you do after your run?
i stretched out and would do some floor work, such as stomach work: sit-ups, leg-raises and crunches (200 each) and push-ups (50 only)

What did you eat for breakfast?
Egg whites, a piece of toast, juice, Gatorade and some vitamins

What time did you go to the gym?
2:00 p.m.

What time did you leave the gym?
4:00 p.m.

What did you do after training?
i would replace my body fluids and have some fruit, then i would go home and rest and relax

What did you eat for dinner?
Chicken, fish and salads (i would have red meat once a week)

What did you do after dinner?
i liked to watch movies, especially the old Charlie Chaplin ones, and i liked music and reading

What time did you go to bed?
9:30 p.m.

What was your favorite exercise?
i liked the speed bag. i liked to hit it so it would spin around, as i thought that was more skilful.

How many days a week did you train?
Six, with Sunday off

Did you have a job before you won the world title?
No

RICARDO LOPEZ'S WORKOUT

WARM-UP	10 minutes of full body stretching 5 minutes of bouncing around on toes while waving arms loosely
SHADOWBOXING	10 minutes
SPARRING	10 x 3 minute rounds (30 second break after each round)
SPEED BAG	8 x 3 minutes (30 second break after each round)
FLOOR-TO-CEILING BAG	3 x 1 minute rounds (30 second break after each round)
STRETCHING	5 minutes
ABDOMINAL WORK	sit-ups leg-raises side-to-sides crunches (500 repetitions of all exercises in total)
NECK EXERCISES	Kneel on the floor with your hands behind your back and your head on a cushion or a mat. Lift your legs and put your hands behind your back so that your body weight is on your head and neck. Rotate your head up and down and from side to side. (Only for the experienced athlete.)
TO FINISH	shower and rest

SVEN OTTKE

What time do you get up?
8:30 a.m.

Do you stretch before your run?
Of course! i'm 37 years old and i need more time for stretching my body.

How far do you run?
i run every second day, between 6 and 7 miles

What do you do after your run?
i stretch my body and then i have a massage. then finish with a steam bath

What do you eat for breakfast?
Some bread, sausage, honey and muesli with nuts

What time do you go to the gym?
Usually in the morning, around 11:30 a.m. for 2–3 hours (3–4 times a week)

What do you do after training?
i finish off with good stretching. Then i go into the sauna, i shower and go home.

What do you eat for dinner?
Before my title fight, i would eat at midday and i would have chicken and pasta. in the evening i would eat nothing

What do you do after dinner?
i like reading and watching TV

What time do you go to bed?
Usually between 10:00 and 11:00 p.m.

What is your favorite exercise?
i love running

How many days a week do you train?
Six or seven days

Did you have a job before you won the world title?
i was a plasterer and later i worked as an industry businessman

SVEN OTTKE'S WORKOUT

WARM-UP	20 minutes of full body stretching
JUMPiNG ROPE	20 minutes (followed by 1 minute break)
HEAVY BAG	6–12 x 3 minute rounds (30 second break after each round), building up as training camp progressed
FOCUS PADS	4–6 x 3 minute rounds, working on combinations (30 second break after each round)
LiGHT WEiGHTS	barbells (with high repetitions) dumbbells (with high repetitions)
FLOOR EXERCISES	sit-ups leg-raises push-ups side-to-sides stretch and hold exercises
WARM-DOWN	full body stretching
TO FiNISH	a walk, then a steam bath

SVEN "THE PHANTOM" OTTKE
IBF and WBA Super Middleweight Champion of the World
Wins 33 **Losses** 0 **Draws** 0
D.O.B.: 06.03.67 **Country born:** Germany

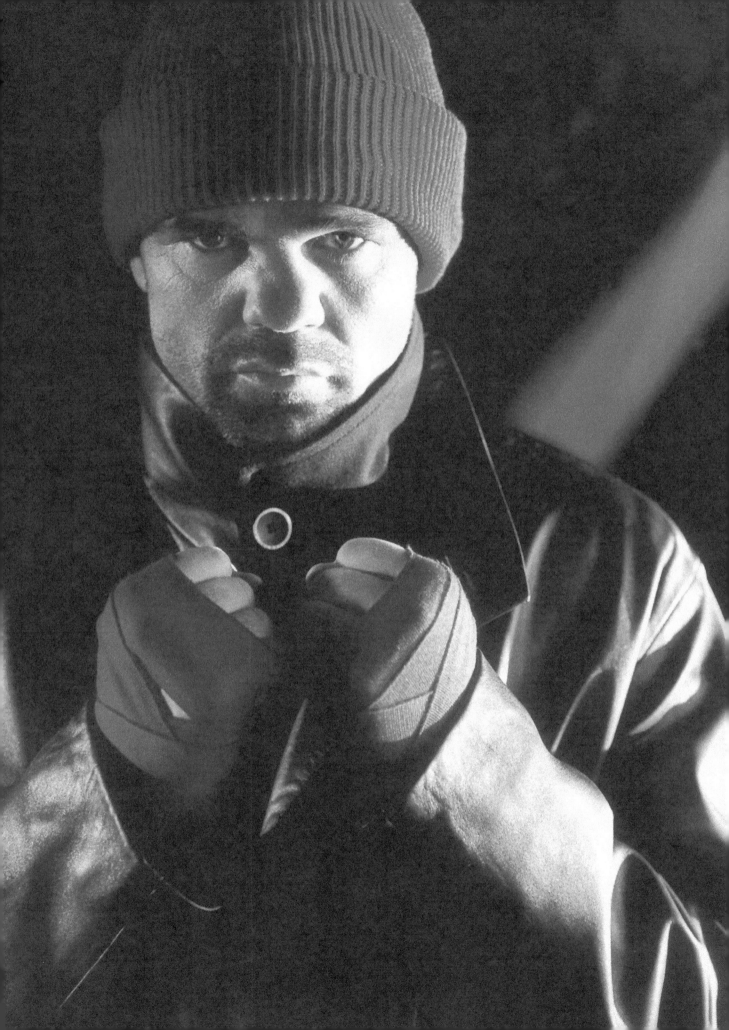

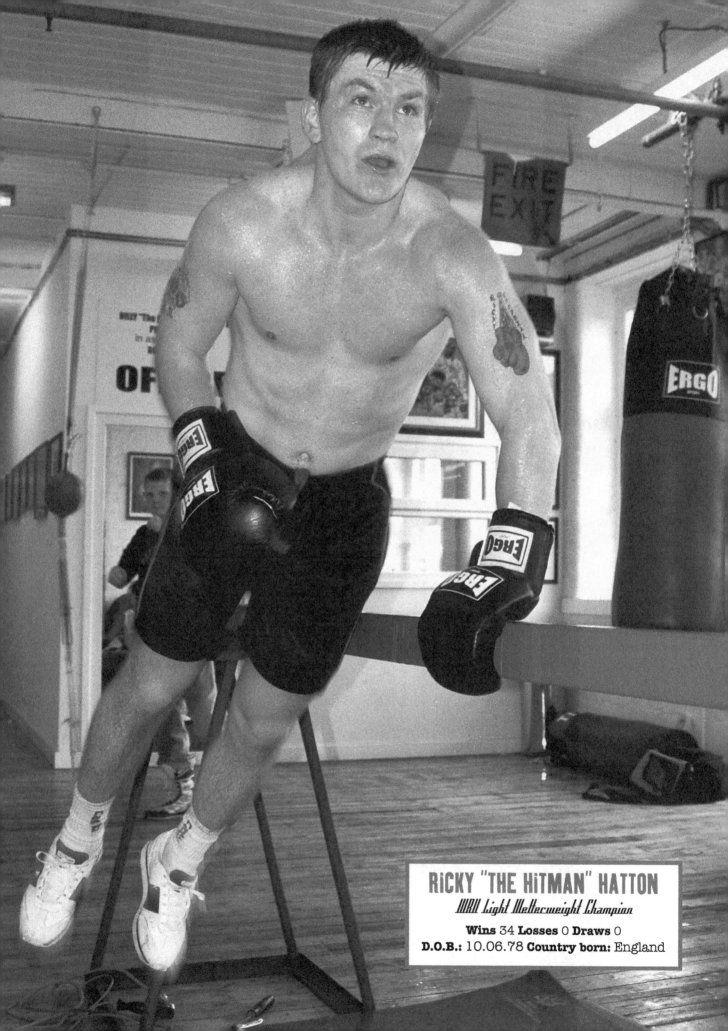

RiCKY "THE HiTMAN" HATTON
WBU Light Welterweight Champion

Wins 34 **Losses** 0 **Draws** 0
D.O.B.: 10.06.78 **Country born:** England

RiCKY HATTON

What time do you get up in the morning?
9:00 a.m.

Do you stretch before you run?
Yes, full stretch and warm-up

How far do you run?
5–6 miles. i run at 7:00 p.m.

After running what do you do?
As it's nighttime, i shower and relax. The reason i run at night is i have a lot more energy for my gym workouts.

What do you have for breakfast?
i have cereal, toast and a cup of tea. On the day of the fight, i have a ritual of going to the local café and having a traditional English breakfast: sausages, eggs, bacon, the lot.

What time do you go to the gym?
12:30 p.m.

What time do you leave the gym?
3:30 p.m., or sometimes later if i am signing autographs for the fans

What do you do after training?
i go home and have something to eat, and relax until it's time to run

What do you eat for dinner?
Chicken, pasta and plenty of vegetables. i also drink lots of mineral water and i take supplements and vitamins.

Do you have any hobbies?
Yes, i love everything to do with boxing and i collect boxing memorabilia. i also love going to see Manchester City football club.

What do you do after your roadwork?
i relax and enjoy playing darts with my dad and my friends

What time do you go to bed?
10:00 p.m.

What is your favorite exercise in the gym?
Bag Bar (*see page 70*)

How many days do you train?
i train in the gym Monday to Friday, and on the weekends i only do roadwork. i train very hard on Monday, Wednesday and Friday; Tuesday and Thursday is still hard (conventional boxing training, floor work, etc.) but not as intense.

Did you have a job before you won the world title?
Yes, i worked in my dad's carpet shop and helped to lay the carpets

RiCKY HATTON'S WORKOUT

WARM-UP	10 minutes full body stretching.
SHADOWBOXiNG	3 x 3 minute rounds (30 second break between each round)
JUMPiNG ROPE	10 minutes non-stop. (Warm-up)
BODY BELT	4–12 x 3 minutes (depending on stage of training camp) Ricky does this exercise working with his trainer. His trainer wears a 6-inch padded leather vest that straps around his body and he uses focus pads. They continuously throw shots at each other. This is the closest thing to fighting, without actually fighting. He also does conventional boxing training (floor work) on alternate days.
BAG BAR	4 x 3 minute rounds (1 minute breaks after each 3 minutes) Ricky uses two pieces of equipment for this exercise: the heavy bag and "the bar," a steel box channel with steel tripod legs at each end (*see page 68*). The bar is about waist-height off the ground, and he starts by jumping over the bar from side to side for 1 minute, then goes to the heavy bag and punches for 1 minute, then back to the bar for 1 minute. Once he gets to the 3 minute mark, he rests. After a break for 1 minute, he repeats the sequence.
STRETCH DOWN	10 minutes
TO FiNiSH	shower and relax

Ricky has a last intense session of training camp one week before the fight.
He always does 15 x 3 minutes on the body belt. He says it's a confidence boost for him.
When he completes this goal, he knows he is ready to fight anyone.

AARON
PRYOR

What time did you get up?
5:00 a.m.

Did you stretch before your run?
Full stretch, which took around 10 minutes

How far did you run?
5 miles

What did you do after your run?
i did some exercises like jumping jacks, sit-ups and press-ups, and finished up with light stretching (15 minutes)

What did you eat for breakfast?
i usually had scrambled eggs, cereal, coffee and water. i would then have a sleep before going to the gym.

What time did you go to the gym?
12:00 midday

What time did you leave the gym?
3:00 p.m.

What did you do after training?
Showered, then i relaxed and maybe watched some TV

What did you eat for dinner?
i had dinner around 5:00 pm. i always had good, nutritious food, like chicken and vegetables, with water and coffee.

What did you do after dinner?
i enjoyed shooting pool and i liked to go for a walk. Before bed i would watch TV.

What time did you go to bed?
9:30 p.m.

What was your favorite exercise?
i liked the heavy bag

How many days a week did you train?
Six days, Sunday off

Did you have a job before you won the world title?
Yes, i worked as a store salesman

AARON PRYOR'S WORKOUT

WARM-UP	20 minutes of full body stretching
SHADOWBOXiNG	3 x 3 minute rounds (30 second break after each round)
LiMBERiNG UP	side-to-sides 3 x 3 minute rounds of bobbing and weaving (30 second break after each round) Bob and weave under a rope attached to the walls at shoulder height, punching upward as you come under the rope and moving forward all the time
SPARRiNG	6–10 x 3 minute rounds (30 second break after each round)
HEAVY BAGS	4 x 3 minute rounds (30 second break after each round)
JUMPiNG ROPE	9 minutes (followed by 30 second break)
FLOOR EXERCISES	25 minutes in total push-ups abdominal work stretching
TO FiNiSH	shower and rest

AARON "THE HAWK" PRYOR
WBA and IBF Light Welterweight Champion of the World
Wins 39 **Losses** 1 **Draws** 0
D.O.B: 10.20.55 **Country born:** U.S.A.

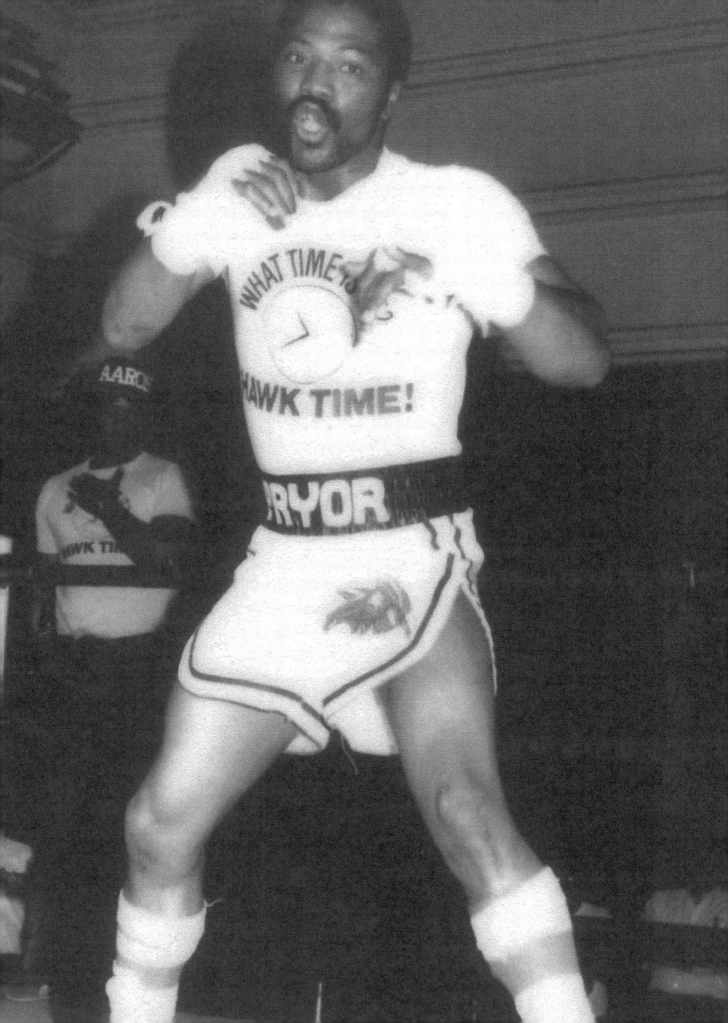

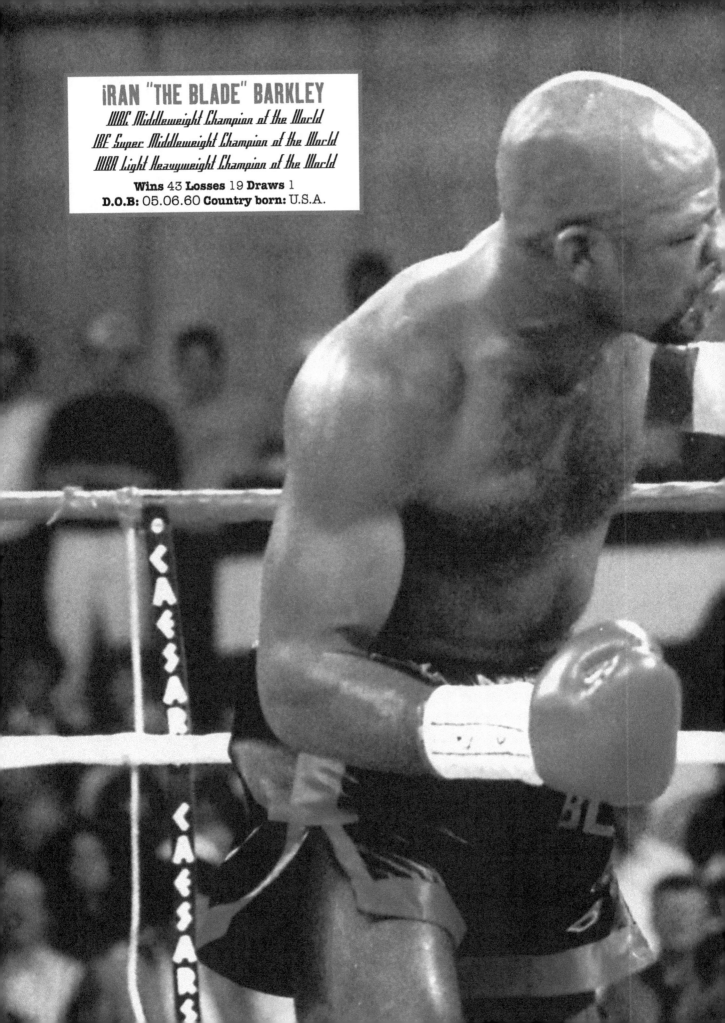

iRAN "THE BLADE" BARKLEY
WBC Middleweight Champion of the World
IBF Super Middleweight Champion of the World
WBA Light Heavyweight Champion of the World

Wins 43 **Losses** 19 **Draws** 1
D.O.B: 05.06.60 **Country born:** U.S.A.

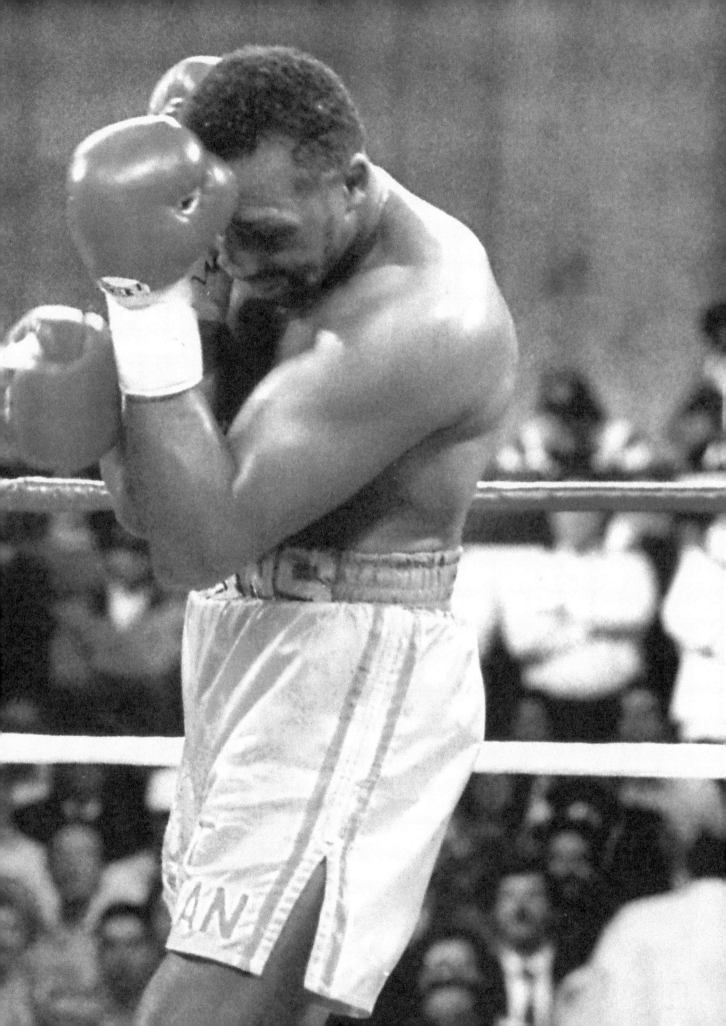

iRAN BARKLEY

What time did you get up?
5:30 a.m.

Did you stretch before your run?
Yes, full stretch

How far did you run?
6 miles

What did you do after your run?
i had a shower and breakfast, then i had a big sleep

What did you eat for breakfast?
Eggs and toast with orange juice

What time did you go to the gym?
5:00 p.m.

What time did you leave the gym?
7:00 p.m.

What did you do after training?
i liked basketball and i watched TV

What did you eat for dinner?
Fish, pasta dishes and vegetables

What did you do after dinner?
i usually had a walk and listened to music

What time did you go to bed?
9:30 p.m.

What was your favorite exercise?
i loved to train, but I didn't have a favorite

How many days a week did you train?
Seven days

Did you have a job before you won the world title?
No

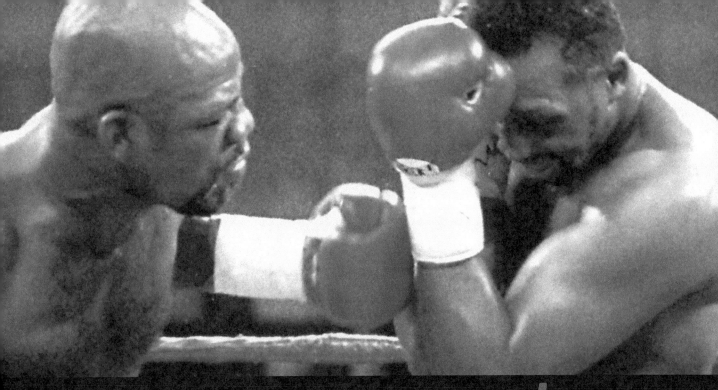

İRAN BARKLEY'S
WORKOUT

WARM-UP	15 minutes of stretching
SPEED BAG	3 x 3 minute rounds (30 second break after each round)
SHADOWBOXING	3 x 3 minute rounds (30 second break after each round)
SPARRING	6 x 3 minute rounds (30 second break after each round)
HEAVY BAG	6–10 x 3 minute rounds (30 second break after each round) iran cut down on heavy bag when sparring
JUMPING ROPE	15 minutes
FLOOR EXERCISES	15 minutes
TO FINISH	massage and steam room, shower and rest

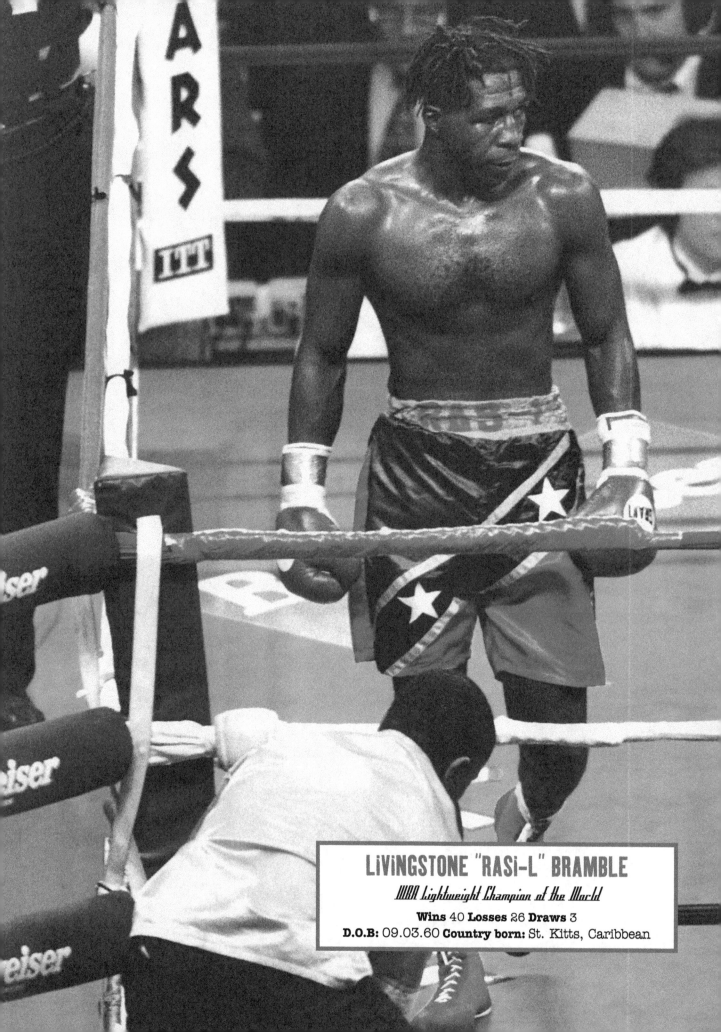

LIVINGSTONE "RASI-L" BRAMBLE
WBA Lightweight Champion of the World
Wins 40 **Losses** 26 **Draws** 3
D.O.B: 09.03.60 **Country born:** St. Kitts, Caribbean

LIVINGSTONE BRAMBLE

What time did you get up?
4:00 a.m.

Did you stretch before your run?
Yes, big stretch

How far did you run?
5–7 miles

What did you do after your run?
i did some exercises, like sit-ups, push-ups and stretching, before going for a walk

What did you eat for breakfast?
i had Quaker Oats oatmeal, fruit juice and water

What time did you go to the gym?
1:30 p.m.

What time did you leave the gym?
4:00 p.m.

What did you do after training?
i liked to go swimming and i loved to dance (jazz dance)

What did you eat for dinner?
Fish or spaghetti

What did you do after dinner?
Relaxed or played golf or basketball

What time did you go to bed?
8:00 p.m.

What was your favorite exercise?
Hitting the heavy bag

How many days a week did you train?
Six days

Did you have a job before you won the world title?
Yes, i worked as a water safety instructor

LIVINGSTONE BRAMBLE'S WORKOUT

WARM-UP	15 minutes of stretching and limbering up
SHADOWBOXiNG	4 x 3 minute rounds (30 second break after each round)
SPARRiNG	4–15 x 3 minute rounds (30 second break after each round) Livingstone built up sparring gradually as his training camp progressed
HEAVY BAG	4 x 3 minute rounds (30 second break after each round)
SPEED BAG	3 x 3 minute rounds (30 second break after each round)
FLOOR-TO-CEiLiNG BAG	3 x 3 minute rounds (30 second break after each round)
JUMPiNG ROPE	12–30 minutes (building up over his training camp)
FLOOR EXERCiSES	2–8 x 25 sit-ups 6 x 25 leg-raises and holds
TO FiNiSH	Livingstone would wrap up in a terry toweling bath robe, lie down and fall asleep for 30 minutes, then have a massage if it was close to the fight, then a shower and rest

JUAN LAPORTE

What time did you get up?
6:00 a.m.

Did you stretch before your run?
Yes, my calves and my sides

How far did you run?
5–6 miles

What did you do after your run?
i shadowboxed and stretched out my body to cool down. i then lay down and had a drink.

What did you eat for breakfast?
Eggs and toast and coffee

What time did you go to the gym?
1:00 p.m.

What time did you leave the gym?
5:00 p.m.

What did you do after training?
i had dinner, then i went for a walk, to walk my dinner off

What did you eat for dinner?
Pasta, fish and occasionally i had steak. i also ate a lot of salads.

What did you do after dinner?
i liked to watch movies

What time did you go to bed?
10:30 p.m.

What was your favorite exercise?
i liked everything, as it all had to be done, but i particularly liked to box and spar

How many days a week did you train?
Six days

Did you have a job before you won the world title?
Yes, i worked in a factory

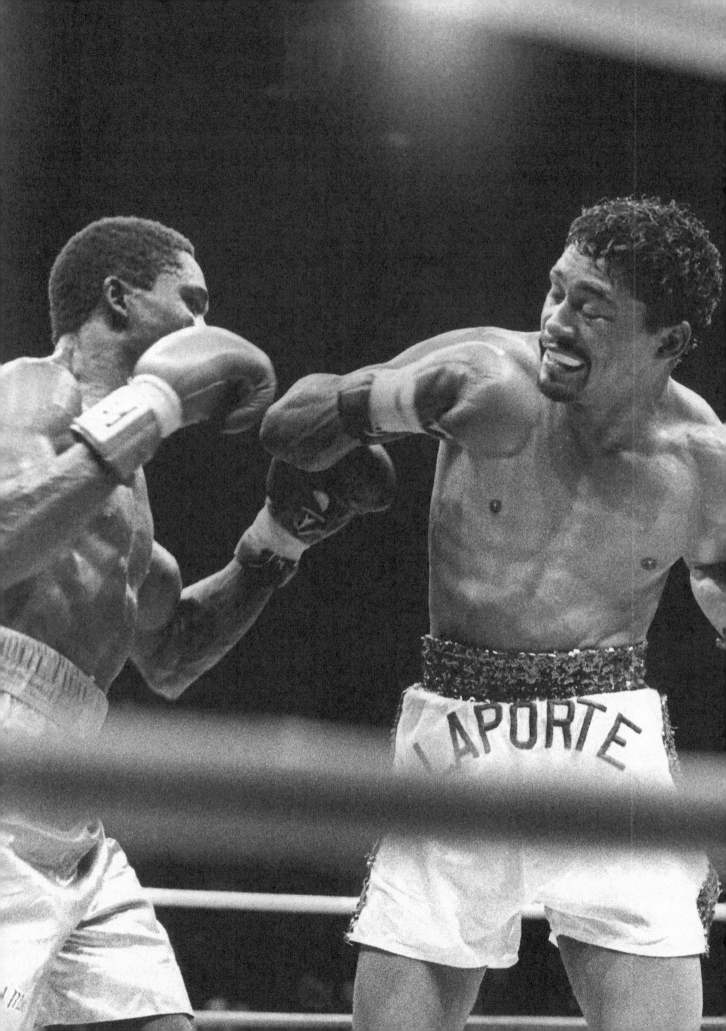

JUAN LAPORTE'S WORKOUT

WARM-UP	15 minutes of loosening up
SHADOWBOXING	6 x 3 minute rounds (30 second break after each round)
SPARRING	5–10 x 3 minute rounds (30 second break after each round) cut down on heavy bag if sparring
HEAVY BAG	6 x 3 minute rounds (30 second break after each round)
JUMPING ROPE	12 minutes (followed by 1 minute break)
FLOOR EXERCISES	200 sit-ups leg-raises 50 press-ups stretching and holding medicine ball exercises (Juan's trainer would mix up the floor exercises so that he never knew what would be next)
TO FINISH	shower and rest

JUAN LAPORTE
WBC Featherweight Champion of the World
Wins 40 **Losses** 17 **Draws** 0
D.O.B: 11.24.59 **Country born:** Puerto Rico

DONALD CURRY

What time did you get up?
6:30 a.m.

How far did you run?
3–5 miles a day, with explosive speed sprinting
on alternate days

What did you do after your run?
i had a rest, then breakfast

What did you eat for breakfast?
Eggs, toast, fruit juice and water

What time did you go to the gym?
it varied. 1:00–3:00 p.m. or 5:00–7:00 p.m.
(2 hours in the gym)

What did you do after training?
i just relaxed and listened to music, or watched a
movie or even played basketball

What did you eat for dinner?
Spaghetti, iced tea, salads

What did you do after dinner?
i liked to read thriller books

What time did you go to bed?
10:00 p.m.

What was your favorite exercise?
i liked to run and i also liked sparring

How many days a week did you train?
Five. Saturday and Sunday were my days off.

Did you have a job before you won the world title?
No

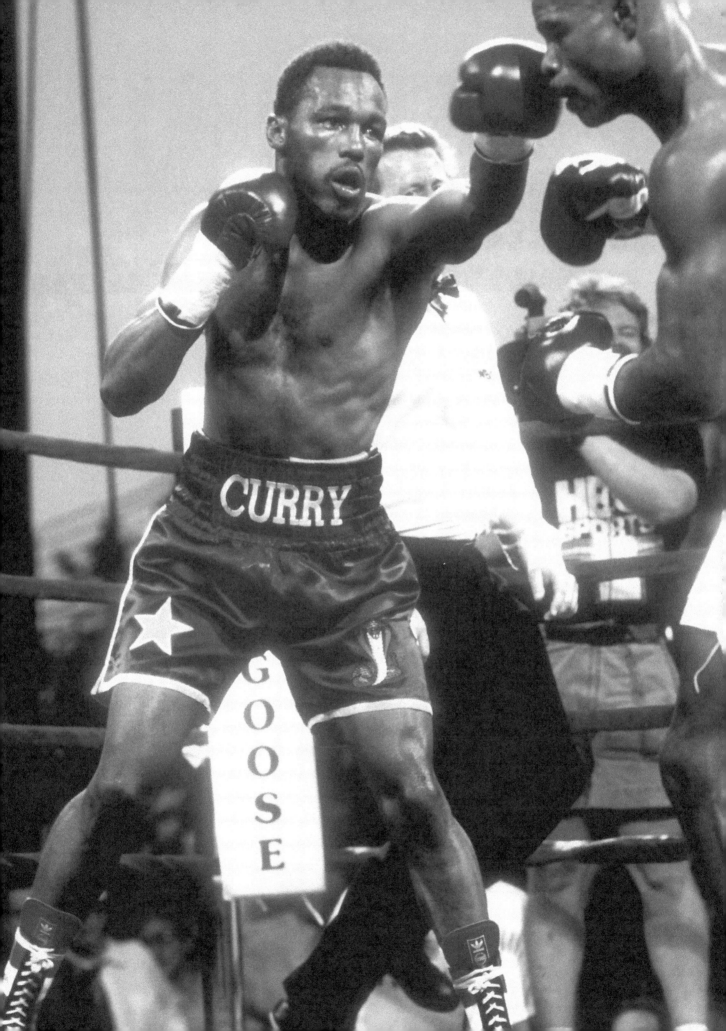

DONALD CURRY'S WORKOUT

WARM-UP	20 minutes of full body stretching
SHADOWBOXiNG	4 x 3 minute rounds (30 second break after each round)
SPARRiNG	4 x 5 minute rounds (30 second break after each round)
FOCUS PADS	4 x 3 minute rounds (30 second break after each round)
FLOOR-TO-CEiLiNG BAG	4 x 3 minute rounds (30 second break after each round)
JUMPiNG ROPE	10 minutes
FLOOR EXERCISES	50 sit-ups 250 leg-raises stomach crunches 80 push-ups 100 side-to-sides
WARM-DOWN	full body stretching
TO FiNiSH	massage and steam room, check weight, then shower and relax

Donald "The Lone Star Cobra" Curry

WBA, IBF and WBC Welterweight Champion of the World
WBC Light Middleweight Champion of the World
Wins 34 **Losses** 6 **Draws** 0
D.O.B.: 09.07.61 **Country born:** U.S.A.

TERRY
NORRiS

What time did you get up?
6:00 a.m.

Did you stretch before your run?
Yes, 20 minute full stretch

How far did you run?
6–8 miles

What did you do after your run?
i went home and had breakfast, then rested

What did you eat for breakfast?
Scrambled eggs, hash browns, orange juice and water

What time did you go to the gym?
Anywhere between 2:30 and 3:30 p.m.

What time did you leave the gym?
i worked out for 2–3 hours each day at the gym, so usually around 6:00 p.m.

What did you do after training?
i liked to go bowling or to the movies, and in the morning i used to play golf

What did you eat for your dinner?
i had pasta dishes, with vegetables on the side

What time did you go to bed?
Around 9:30 p.m.

What was your favorite exercise?
i loved hitting the floor-to-ceiling bag

How many days a week did you train?
Six, with Sunday off

Did you have a job before you won the world title?
No

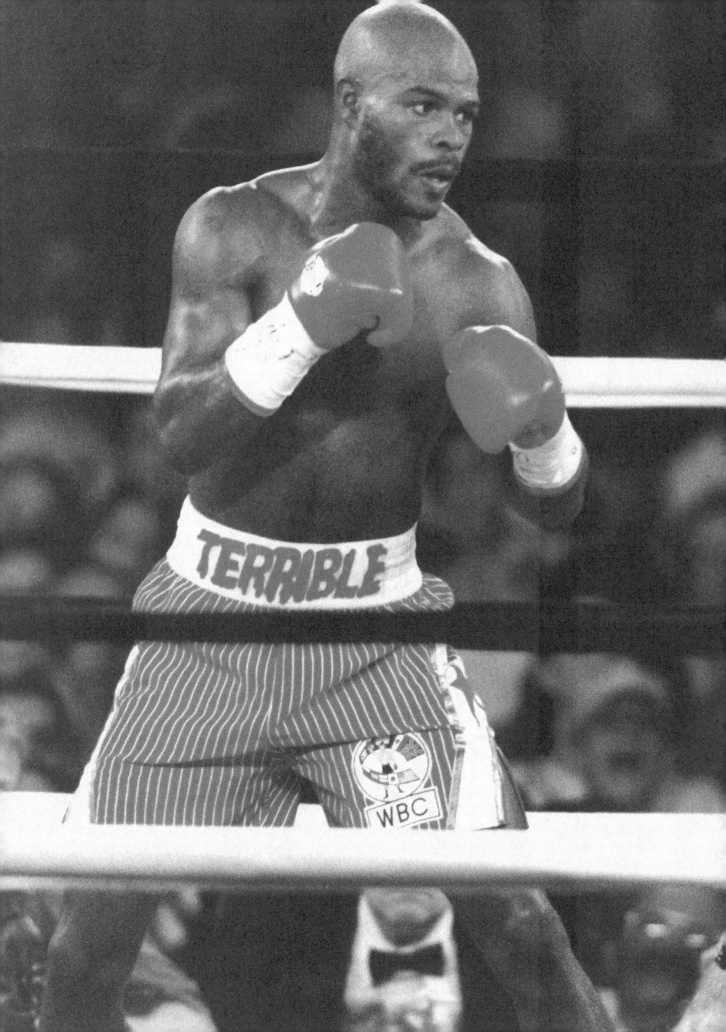

TERRY NORRIS' WORKOUT

WARM-UP	20 minutes of full body stretching
SHADOWBOXING	4 x 3 minute rounds (30 second break after each round)
SPARRING	12 x 3 minute rounds (30 second break after each round) Terry worked up to this level over a six-week training camp
FLOOR-TO-CEILING BAG	4 x 3 minutes (30 second break after each round)
HEAVY BAG	4 x 3 minute rounds (30 second break after each round)
JUMPING ROPE	12 minutes
WARM-DOWN	5 minutes
TO FINISH	rest, massage, shower and rest

Terry "Terrible" Norris
WBA, WBC and IBF Light Middleweight Champion of the World
Wins 47 **Losses** 9 **Draws** 0
D.O.B.: 06.16.67 **Country born:** U.S.A.

MATTHEW SAAD MUHAMMAD

What time did you get up?
4:30 a.m.

Did you stretch before your run?
Yes, 20 minutes

How far did you run?
3 miles

What did you do after your run?
i did some exercises, then i jumped rope and
finished off with stretching

What did you eat for breakfast?
Poached eggs, bread, fruit juice

What time did you go to the gym?
4:00 p.m.

What time did you leave the gym?
6:30–7:00 p.m.

What did you do after training?
i had to do promotional work and i also liked to
help out the kids

What did you eat for dinner?
i liked steak or veal, with vegetables or salad
on the side

What did you do after dinner?
i liked to play chess, and watch and play basketball

What time did you go to bed?
10:00 p.m.

What was your favorite exercise?
i liked to jump rope

How many days a week did you train?
Five, with Saturday and Sunday off

Did you have a job before you won the world title?
Yes, i was a construction worker. i enjoyed the hard
work, because i treated it like training.

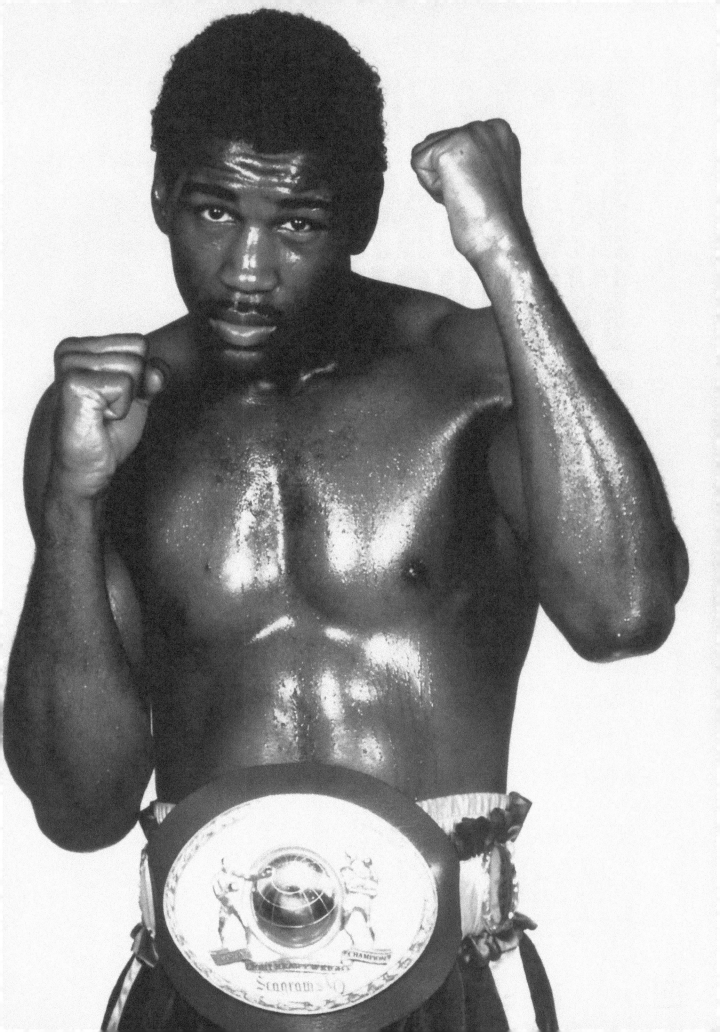

MATTHEW SAAD MUHAMMAD'S WORKOUT

WARM-UP	20 minutes of full body stretching
JUMPING ROPE	24 minutes
SPEED BAG	4–6 x 3 minute rounds (30 second break after each round)
HEAVY BAG	4 x 3 minute rounds (30 second break after each round)
SPARRING	depending on progress in training camp
LIGHT WEIGHTS	high repetitions at fast rate
TREADMILL	30 minutes
SHADOWBOXING	6 x 3 minute rounds (30 second break after each round)
JUMPING ROPE	12 minutes
TO FINISH	wrap up with towel and cool down, steam room, shower

Matthew Saad Muhammad
WBC Light Heavyweight Champion of the World
Wins 39 **Losses** 16 **Draws** 3
D.O.B.: 06.16.54 **Country born:** U.S.A.

MiKE
MCCALLUM

What time did you get up?
5:00 a.m.

Did you stretch before your run?
Yes

How far did you run?
4 miles

What did you do after your run?
i would have breakfast, then i would rest

What did you eat for breakfast?
Two eggs, toast, fruit juice, and i enjoyed a cup
of tea

What time did you go to the gym?
1:00 p.m.

What time did you leave the gym?
3:00 p.m.

What did you do after training?
i would relax, and i liked playing table tennis

What did you eat for dinner?
Fish or chicken with salads

What did you do after dinner?
i watched TV and videotapes of the guy i was fighting

What time did you go to bed?
9:00 p.m.

What was your favorite exercise?
Sparring

How many days a week did you train?
Six days

Did you have a job before you won the world title?
No

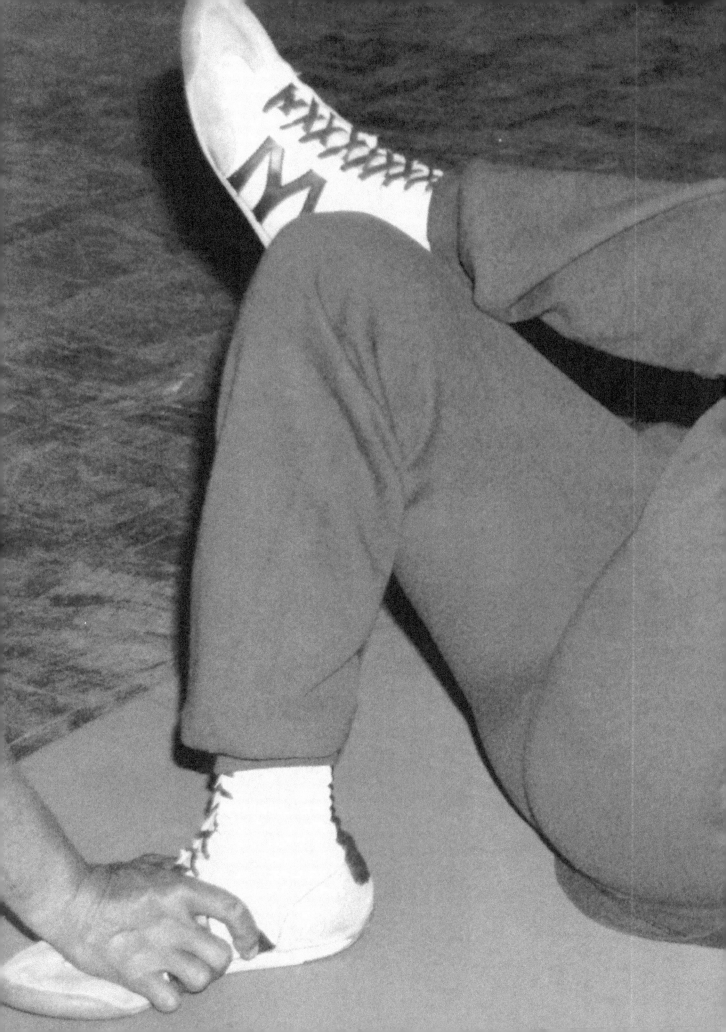

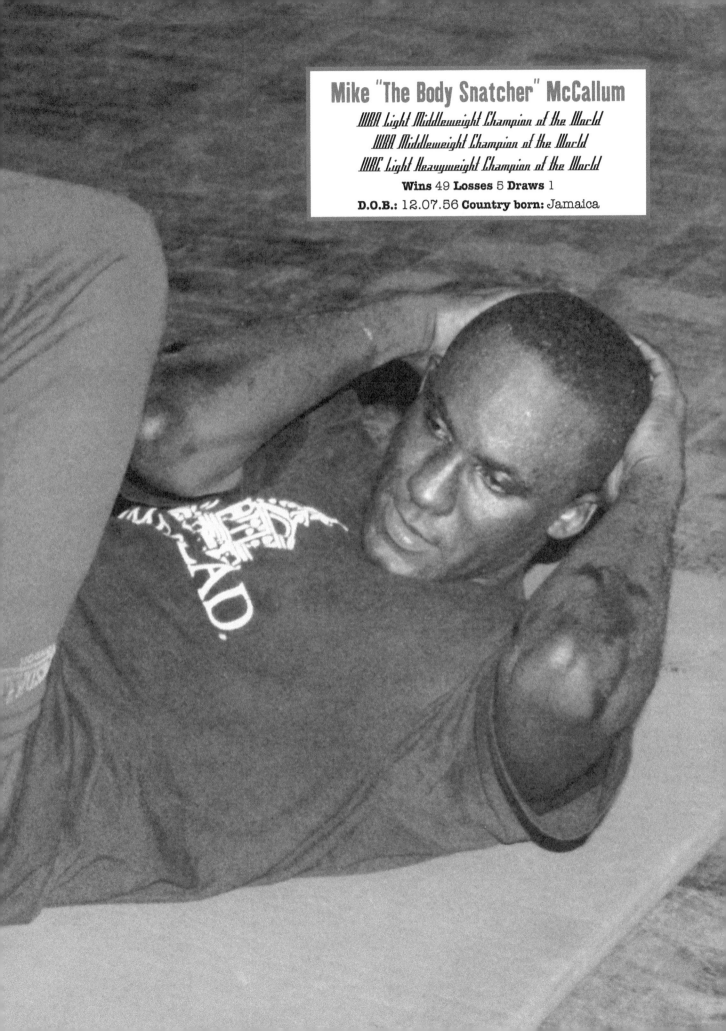

Mike "The Body Snatcher" McCallum
WBA Light Middleweight Champion of the World
WBA Middleweight Champion of the World
WBC Light Heavyweight Champion of the World
Wins 49 **Losses** 5 **Draws** 1
D.O.B.: 12.07.56 **Country born:** Jamaica

MIKE McCALLUM'S WORKOUT

WARM-UP	20 minutes of full body stretching
SHADOWBOXING	3 x 3 minute rounds (30 second break after each round)
HEAVY BAG	4 x 3 minute rounds (30 second break after each round)
SPARRING	6–12 x 3 minute rounds (30 second break after each round) (Mike would build up his sparring as his training camp progressed)
SPEED BAG	3 minutes (followed by 30 second break)
JUMPING ROPE	15 minutes (followed by 30 second break)
FLOOR EXERCISES	25 minutes in total sit-ups leg-raises push-ups stretches and holds for 1 minute (Mike's trainer used to mix it up so that he would never know which exercise would be next)
TO FINISH	massage (depending on how he felt), then shower and rest

CHRISTY MARTIN

What time do you get up?
7:00 a.m. I have breakfast, then get ready for the gym. I train in the morning and run in the evening.

What do you eat for breakfast?
A lot of protein, such as eggs and bacon, and water

What time do you go to the gym?
10:00 a.m.

What time do you leave the gym?
1:00 p.m.

What do you do after training?
I like to swim and I love riding my Harley Davidson motorcycle

What do you eat for dinner?
Dinner is usually chicken and salads or sometimes I'll have steak (no rice or potatoes)

What do you do after dinner?
I hang around and relax, then I get mentally prepared to run

Do you stretch before your run?
Yes, light stretching

How far do you run?
3–4 miles, and I also incorporate explosive sprinting into my running

What do you do after your run?
I walk around to cool down, then I shower and unwind for the rest of the night

What time do you go to bed?
I'm a night owl, and I don't usually go to bed until 1:30 a.m.

What is your favorite exercise?
Focus pads

How many days a week do you train?
Six days on and Sunday off

Did you have a job before you won the world title?
Yes, I was a school teacher

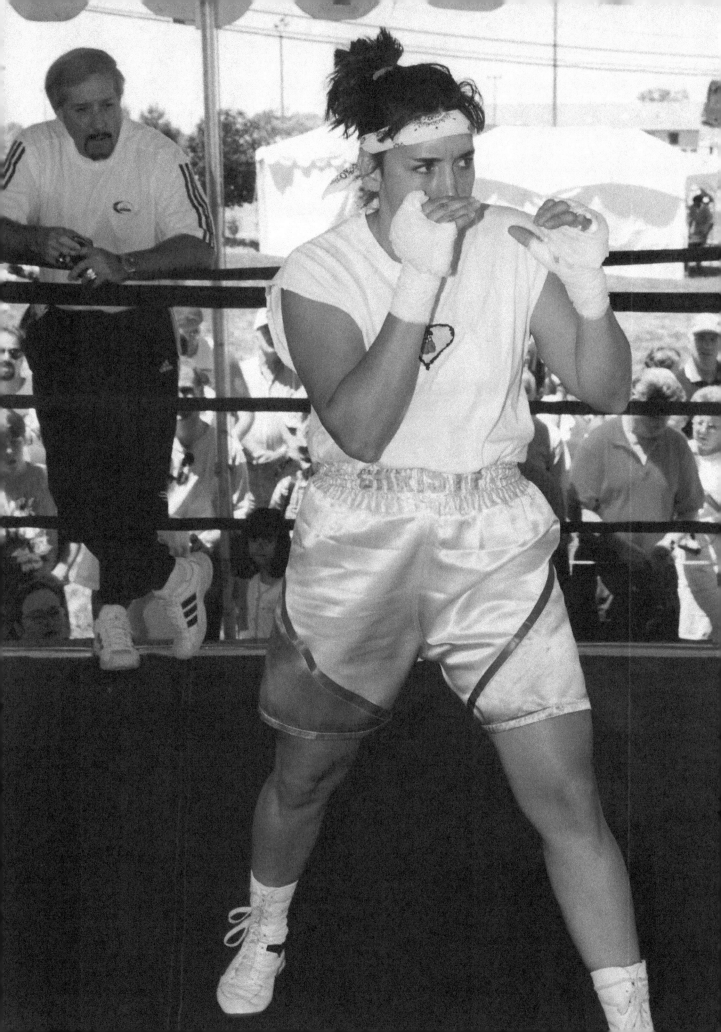

CHRISTY MARTIN'S WORKOUT

WARM-UP	10 minutes of light stretching
SHADOWBOXING	3 x 3 minute rounds (1 minute break after each round)
HEAVY BAG	4 x 3 minute rounds (1 minute break after each round)
FLOOR-TO-CEILING BAG	2 x 3 minute rounds (1 minute break after each round)
FOCUS PADS	3 x 3 minute rounds (1 minute break after each round)
SPEED BAG	3 x 3 minute rounds (1 minute break after each round)
JUMPING ROPE	12 minutes
FLOOR EXERCISES	100 sit-ups 50 leg-raises 100 crunches 15 push-ups
TO FINISH	shower and rest

Christy "The Coalminer's Daughter" Martin
Women's Welterweight Champion of the World
Wins 45 **Losses** 3 **Draws** 2
D.O.B.: 06.12.68 **Country born:** U.S.A.

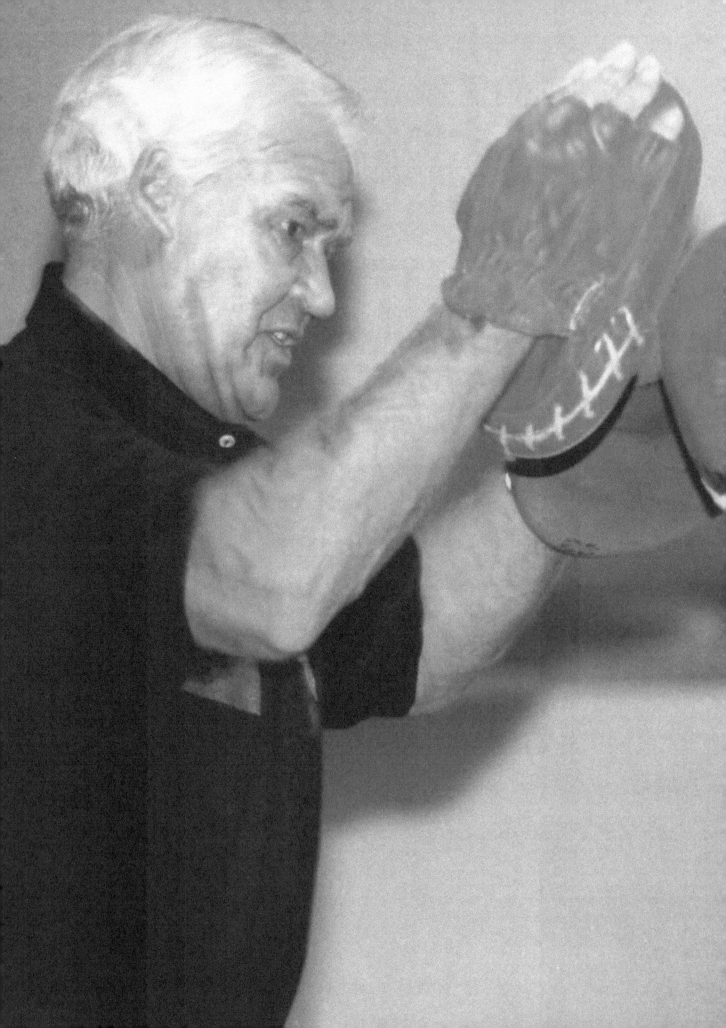

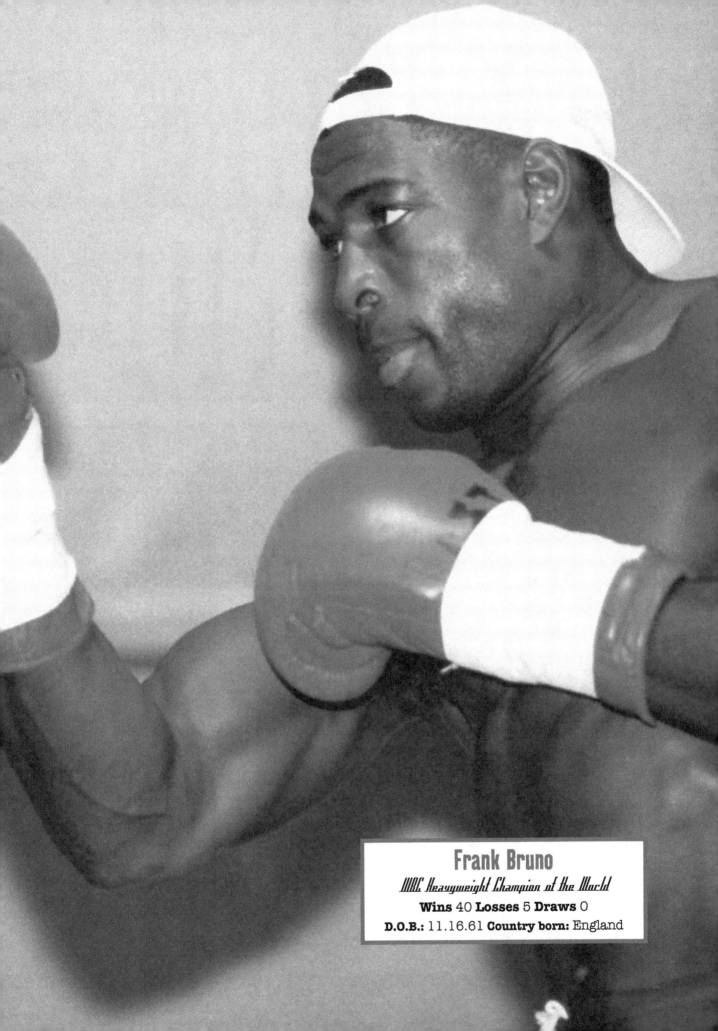

Frank Bruno
WBC Heavyweight Champion of the World
Wins 40 **Losses** 5 **Draws** 0
D.O.B.: 11.16.61 **Country born:** England

FRANK BRUNO

What time did you get up?
6:00 a.m., for a 6:30 a.m. run

Did you stretch before your run?
Yes, full body stretch, which takes up to 15 minutes

How far did you run?
Usually 5–6 miles. i also had a few hills on my run route, which i sprinted up then eased off when i reached the top.

What did you do after your run?
i always jumped rope for 6 minutes, then i would do some stretching and calisthenics. Then George Francis would make me take a cold plunge in the outside pond.

What did you eat for breakfast?
Fruit juice, cereal, some fruit and yogurt, and plenty of water

What did you do after breakfast?
i went for a walk and then i would have a lie down. i also fitted in my charity and promotional work. Then i had my lunch around midday.

What time did you go to the gym?
i would go at around 2:30 p.m. for a massage before i did my gym work

What time did you leave the gym?
5:30 p.m. i always finished with a massage, then a shower, and home for my dinner.

What did you eat for dinner?
Always healthy, nutritious food: chicken, rice, veggies, pasta, fruit, and plenty of water. The most important thing is to have a balanced diet.

What did you do after dinner?
i used to go for a walk, then i would watch the TV or read. i also like my music.

What time did you go to bed?
10:00 p.m.

What was your favorite exercise?
it all had to be done!

How many days a week did you train?
Five days, and a light run on Saturday morning. i had Sunday off.

Did you have a job before you won the world title?
i had a few. i worked as a barman in a bingo hall.

FRANK BRUNO'S WORKOUT

WARM-UP

15–20 minutes full body stretching

SHADOWBOXING

3 x 3 minute rounds working on combinations (30 second break after each round)

HEAVY BAG

4 x 3 minute rounds (30 second break after each round)
(Frank sometimes substituted sparring for the heavy bag)

FOCUS PADS

3 x 3 minute rounds working on combinations, or trying new ones
(30 second break after each round)

SPEED BAG

3 x 3 minute rounds (30 second break after each round)

STATIONARY BIKE

18 minutes (listening to Walkman)

MACHINE GYMWORK

seated chest press, out from shoulders, in and out at fast pace
cable machine, alternating hands out, at fast pace
light weights, high reps at fast pace
pull-down cable machine
seated shoulder press up above head at fast pace

ABDOMINAL EXERCISES

100 side-to-sides
3 x 20 leg-raises with medicine ball (30 second break after each set)
3 x 20 medicine ball drops (30 second break after each set)
sit-up/stand-ups (*see Nigel Benn's workout, page 33*)

Medicine Ball

HOW TO: Lie on your back with a trainer standing over you. Get your trainer to drop a medicine ball onto your stomach. Tense up the muscles in your stomach and push off the ball with your hands, back to your trainer. Continue to let the ball hit your stomach until you finish your repetitions. Do this at moderate to fast pace.

WEIGHTS

Frank hangs weights from a specially designed head strap. Once the weight is hooked on, he raises and lowers his head to build up his neck and shoulder muscles.

TO FINISH

walk around, have a drink, then a massage

CHARLIE MAGRi

What time did you get up?
6:00 a.m.

Did you stretch before your run?
Yes, full body stretch

How far did you run?
5 miles

What did you do after your run?
i stretched out again, then i rugged up with a towel over my head and sweated out

What did you eat for breakfast?
Poached eggs, toast, fresh orange juice and water. i then had a rest before i went to the gym.

What time did you go to the gym?
12:00 midday

What time did you leave the gym?
3:00 p.m.

What did you do after training?
i went home and took my dogs for a walk, then i relaxed

What did you eat for dinner?
i had salads, steak and fish

What did you do after dinner?
i usually went for a walk and i watched soccer on the TV

What time did you go to bed?
11:00 p.m.

What was your favorite exercise?
i loved jumping rope

How many days a week did you train?
Six days, with Saturdays off to watch the soccer

Before you won the world title, did you have a job?
Yes, i worked as a tailor's cloth-cutter

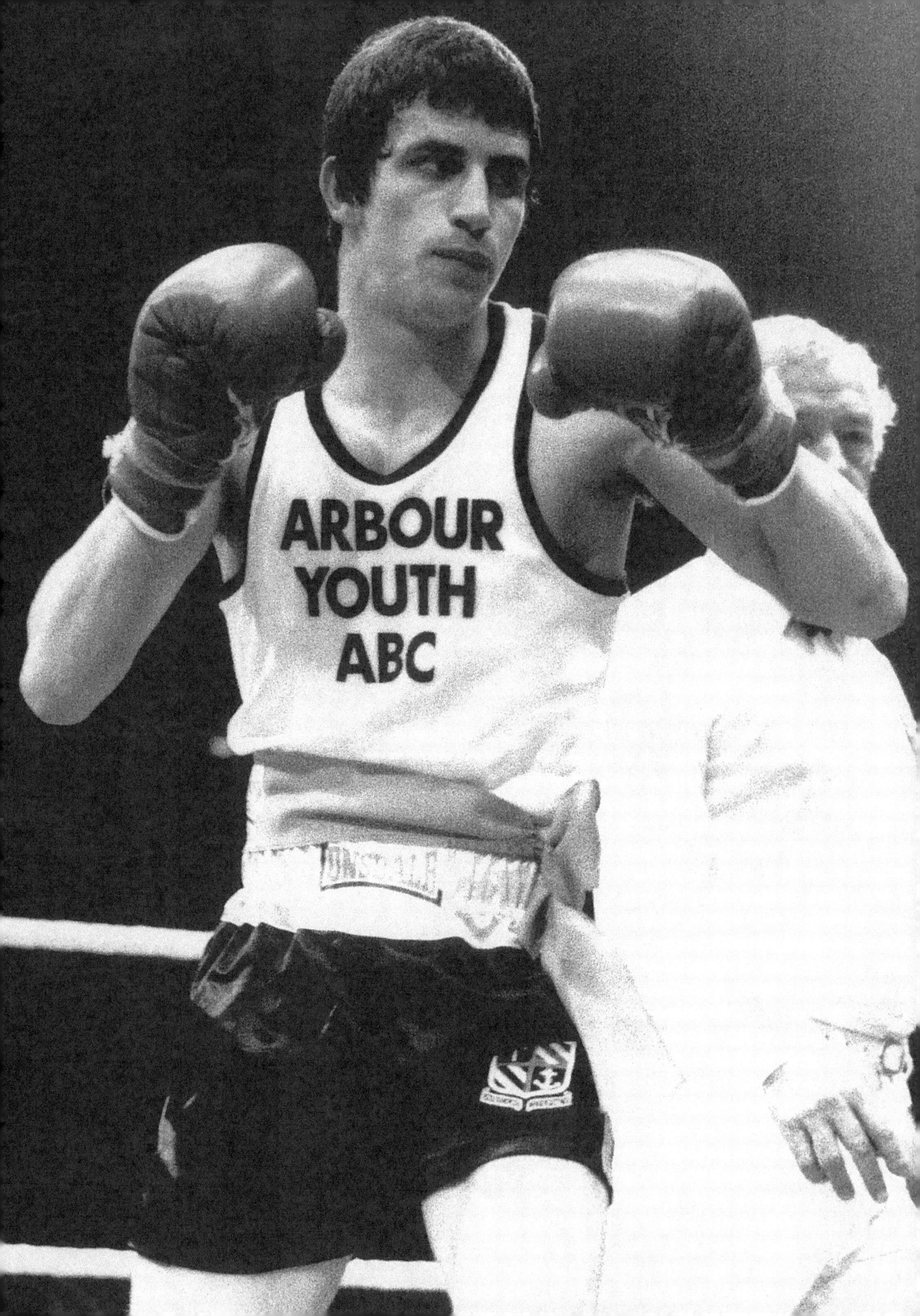
ARBOUR
YOUTH
ABC

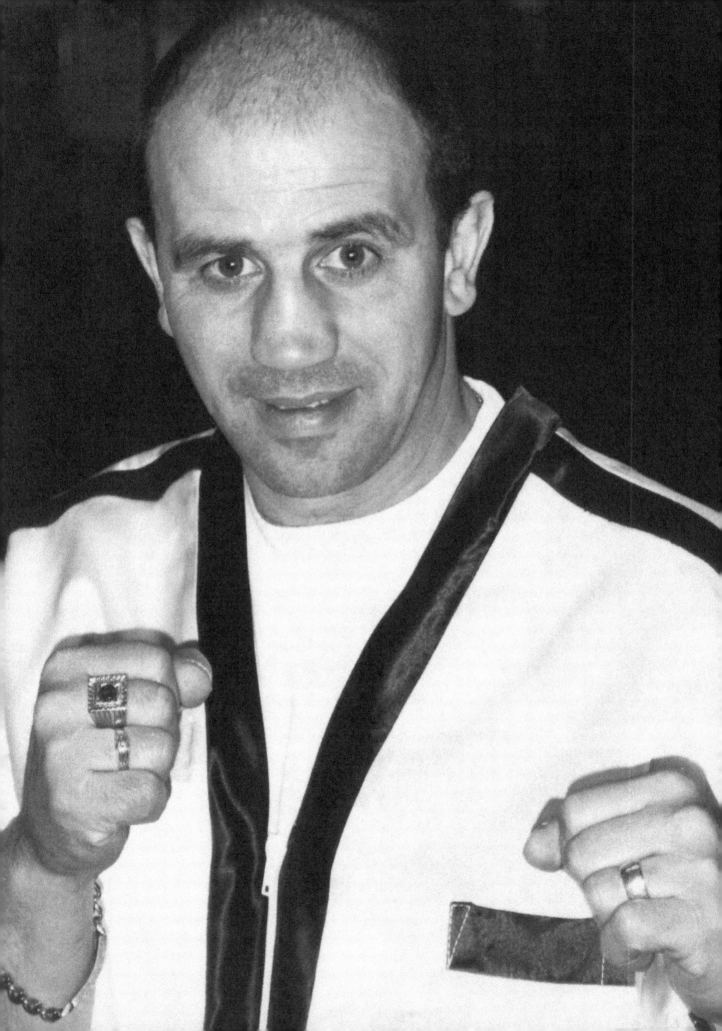

CHARLIE MAGRI'S WORKOUT

WARM-UP	10 minutes of full body stretching
SHADOWBOXING	5 x 3 minute rounds (30 second break after each round)
SPARRING	8 x 3 minute rounds (30 second break after each round)
HEAVY BAG	2 x 3 minute rounds (30 second break after each round)
STATIONARY BIKE	15 minutes
FLOOR EXERCISES	10 x 15 sit-ups 10 x 15 leg-raises
STRETCH OUT	5–10 minutes
SHADOWBOXING	3 minutes
TO FINISH	sweat out wrapped up tightly in towel, then shower

CHARLIE MAGRI
WBC Flyweight Champion of the World
Wins 30 **Losses** 5 **Draws** 0
D.O.B.: 07.20.56 **Country born:** England

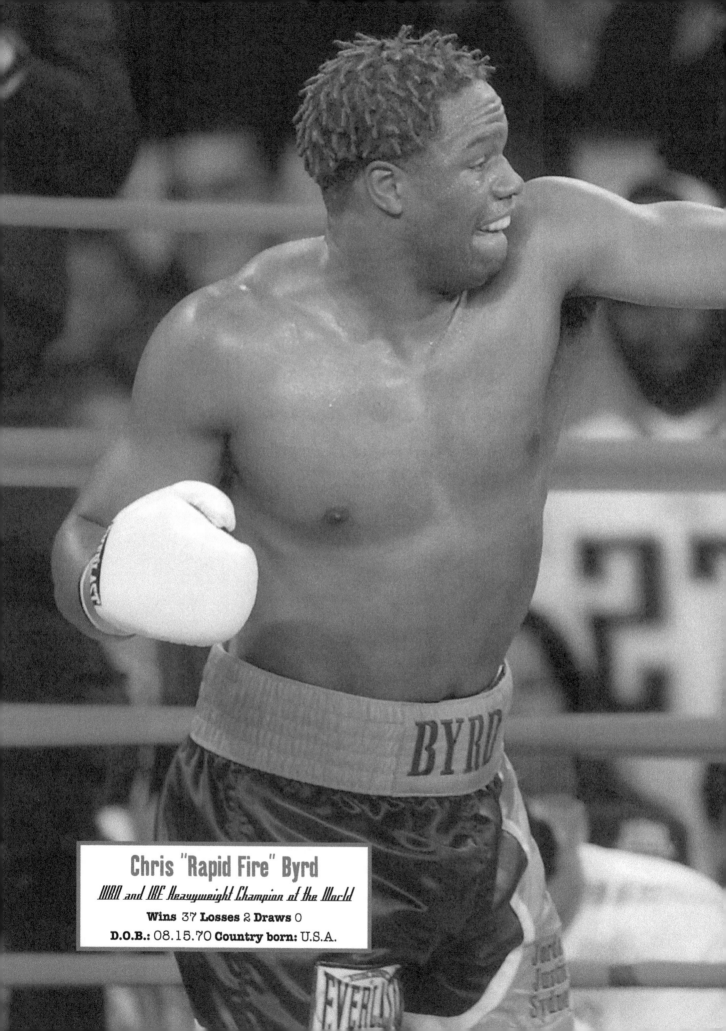

Chris "Rapid Fire" Byrd

WBO and IBF Heavyweight Champion of the World

Wins 37 **Losses** 2 **Draws** 0

D.O.B.: 08.15.70 **Country born:** U.S.A.

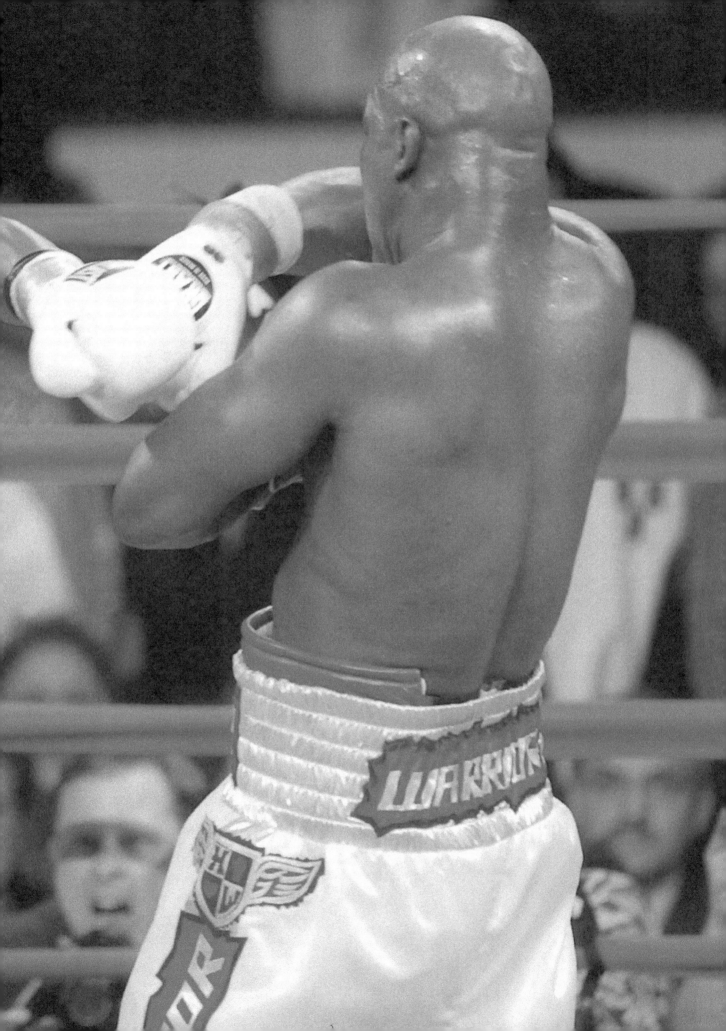

CHRIS BYRD

What time do you get up?
5:30 a.m.

Do you stretch before your run?
Yes, full stretch out

How far do you run?
5 miles. i incorporate high-elevation hill runs and sprints into my run.

What do you do after your run?
i rest my body and get prepared for my workout. i also have some breakfast.

What do you eat for breakfast?
i have fruit, cereal, oatmeal and orange juice

What time do you go to the gym?
1:00 p.m.

What time do you leave the gym?
3:30–4:00 p.m.

What do you do after training?
i go home and relax. i like to play Nintendo or PlayStation 2 and i also read my Bible every day.

What do you eat for dinner?
i usually have pasta, chicken and some vegetables

What do you do after dinner?
i like watching basketball and football, and i love spending time with my family

What time do you go to bed?
10:00–10:30 p.m.

What is your favorite exercise?
i love to jump rope

How many days a week do you train?
Six, with Sundays off

Did you have a job before you won the world title?
No, i've always been a boxer

CHRIS BYRD'S WORKOUT

WARM-UP	full body stretching
SHADOWBOXING	6 x 3 minute rounds (30 second break after each round)
HEAVY BAG	6 x 3 minute rounds, working on combinations (30 second drilling the heavy bag after each round, 30 second break only)
FLOOR-TO-CEILING BAG	3 x 3 minute rounds (30 second break after each round)
JUMPING ROPE	20 minutes
FLOOR EXERCISES	sit-ups medicine ball exercises stretching
TO FINISH	hot tub, rub-down/massage and shower

MY
WORK

OUT WORKOUT

ACTION PLAN

The idea to write this section came to me one day after I had just finished my workout. I'm a creature of habit and always have the same routine when I get to the changing room. I have a drink, I sit on the bench and kind of meditate, letting my mind wander. On this particular day I got to thinking how hard it is for the average person (like me) to fit in all their commitments and still manage consistently good, hard workouts. Rushing from work to catch a fitness class while juggling other commitments is not easy. My solution: ditch the classes and train whenever I found the time, rather than commit to someone else's timetable.

I've devised the following program because I know there must be others with the same time problems. Whenever you can find the 30, 60 or 90 minutes required for these workouts then you can just get straight into it. Having a structured exercise regime is really important. Just turning up to the gym and mindlessly bashing away at a bag is a sure recipe for staleness and boredom. My program has two basic components: roadwork and gym and boxing work.

Now, some of you will be thinking, "Well, that's all very well, Gary, but I simply don't have time, what with work and family and everything else." To this I say, respectfully: you *must* find the time. You can't tell me you can't find *one* morning, *one* lunch hour, *one* after-work and *one* hour on the weekend? Think of it like this: a healthy you is a happy you, which is a good thing for your family, friends, workmates, everyone — you, most particularly. Working out is an investment in your own well-being, an investment in your quality of life. What could be more important?

DREAMS AND GOALS

Apart from being particularly good at boxing, the boxers in this book are the same as you. They are motivated to get up in the morning to chase their dreams; theirs just happen to be world titles rather than a fishing boat or a holiday in Disneyland. We all have dreams and goals. It's important to have something to work and strive toward. Having a dream can keep you positive in life, which is all that really matters. My advice: set yourself a realistic goal, write down the steps that you need to pass to achieve the goal, stick it on the fridge or somewhere to remind yourself, then go out and do it! You are the only one who can set yourself a goal in life and make it happen. Do it right now!

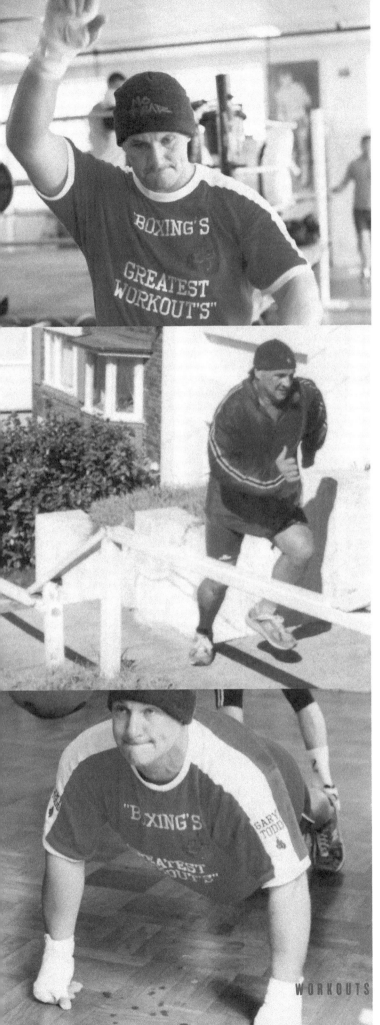

EATiNG RiGHT

The merits of the nutritional value of certain foods in a training regime is a whole other book, but it nearly goes without saying that when you're training, it's essential to eat good, healthy food. Here are a few other reminders:

1 Never eat just before bed.

2 Drink plenty of water. Try to drink 8–12 glasses a day — your body needs a lot of water, especially if you are doing heavy workouts. And always have a drink of water before bed — your body needs it, and you'll feel more energized when you wake up. Eight hours is a long time without a drink.

3 Try to eat one portion of protein, one of carbohydrates, and at least one of vegetables for lunch and dinner.

4 Give yourself a break once a week and eat whatever you fancy.

5 Train on an empty stomach and have your last meal 2–3 hours before your workout.

6 Watch portion sizes. The key to losing weight is to burn more calories than you consume — hard to do when you're wolfing a bucket of fried chicken every other day.

7 Eat in moderation. Try to eat 5–6 small meals a day, rather than three whoppers.

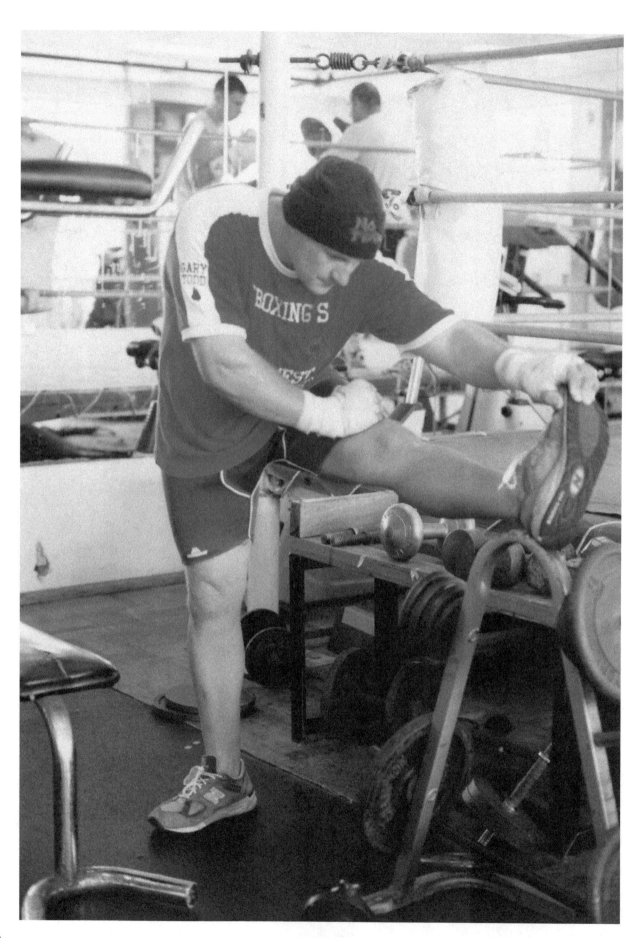

ROADWORK

Running has many benefits that will help improve your all-around fitness, not just your boxing. It develops cardio-vascular efficiency, raises your VO$_2$ max, keeps your joints strong and clears your head by burning off stress hormones. You don't have to start out at a cracking pace. Begin by alternating a few minutes of running with a few minutes of walking, gradually extending the length of time that you spend running. You'll soon see and feel the results.

R unning and jogging should definitely be the most important part of your fitness plan. I cannot stress enough how important it is for your body and your legs that you run. It's probably not going to be the most enjoyable aspect of your training regime at first, but I promise that if you persevere, then you'll soon be seeing much better results in the gym. Over the years I've seen guys who didn't like doing roadwork take the easy way out by doing weights or jumping on the bike machine. Those who did their roadwork and persevered nearly always went on to show impressive results. The guys who didn't just floated around and didn't step up to the next level.

How to start

Like everything, it takes time to build up your stints out on the road, so don't worry if you're not running as well as you thought you might. It will come together for you at some point. What you have to do is start out jogging and listen to your body. You will hear your heart thumping and your breath blowing in and out. When I run I hear these sounds and I work them into each step. Once you get this right, you can get into a steady rhythm and build on it. Getting into a rhythm is the key. Your body will tell you if you're going too quickly and not breathing in time because you'll get a stitch. Don't worry: if this does happen, you just have to slow it down a bit and get your breathing right.

Another reason some people don't like to run is that they say it's boring. Everyone is different, but what I like to do is consider what I've done that day (I generally run after work) or what's coming up tomorrow. Running is a great head-clearer, and I often have some of my best ideas three-quarters of the way through. These days, my training runs last about 40 minutes — or 20 minutes if I am doing sprint or hill work. Another good way to fight boredom is to stick a headset on. I have a tape with my favorite training songs on it. You might want to listen to a book on tape or a football game. Favorite songs or your team winning will definitely help you get up that steep hill or finish strongly.

STRETCHING

I always stretch before I start my run. Some boxers don't bother, but it's a fact that stretching is good for you. It warms and loosens the muscles, improves their range of motion and prepares them for effort.

Simply put, inflexible, cold muscles are not able to do what warm, loose muscles can. Without a proper warm-up you risk muscle soreness at best — or even torn muscles, which can keep you from training.

I usually do toe-touches (holding for 10 seconds), leg stretches and torso twists. Remember: always breathe normally when you are holding a stretch. Listen to your body — it will tell you when you have done enough.

Getting out there

It's very important that you run on an empty stomach. The time of day you're running will obviously dictate when you will have had your last meal. If you run in the early morning, that's easy — have your breakfast after that. If you run in the afternoon — let's say 5 p.m. — then you should have a snack around 2 p.m. (A banana, an apple or a cracker and a drink will see you through until 5 p.m.) However, if you are hungry — eat. Never intentionally miss out on a meal. It does your body no good. Your body needs fuel to work.

Okay, it's time to get going. You've done your stretching, had a drink, used the restroom and you have an idea of where you want to go. Start off slowly, get into your stride and incorporate this into your breathing. It takes about 10–15 minutes to get into your stride and to get your body to the right temperature.

Another useful thing to do is time yourself. Get yourself a small stopwatch or just use a wristwatch. You'll hear a lot of people counting the

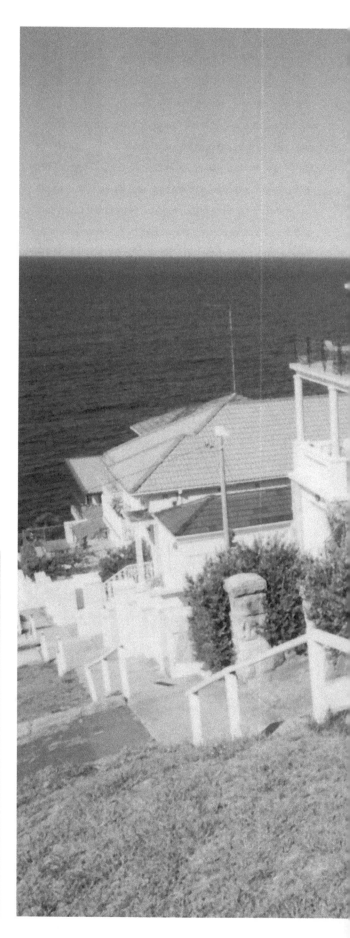

HiLL WORK

Including hills or steep steps into your run can give you a great buzz and a real sense of achievement. Use these tips to help you push through to the end.

1 As you approach your hill, take a big breath and blow out. Start climbing, pacing yourself and looking down at the ground. Remember not to look up — it's hard enough, without having to see what you still have to run up!

2 When you start to climb, pump your arms back and forth to help you get up.

3 Try not to stop when you reach the top. Keep jogging and get back into your normal pace. Your breathing will also stabilize.

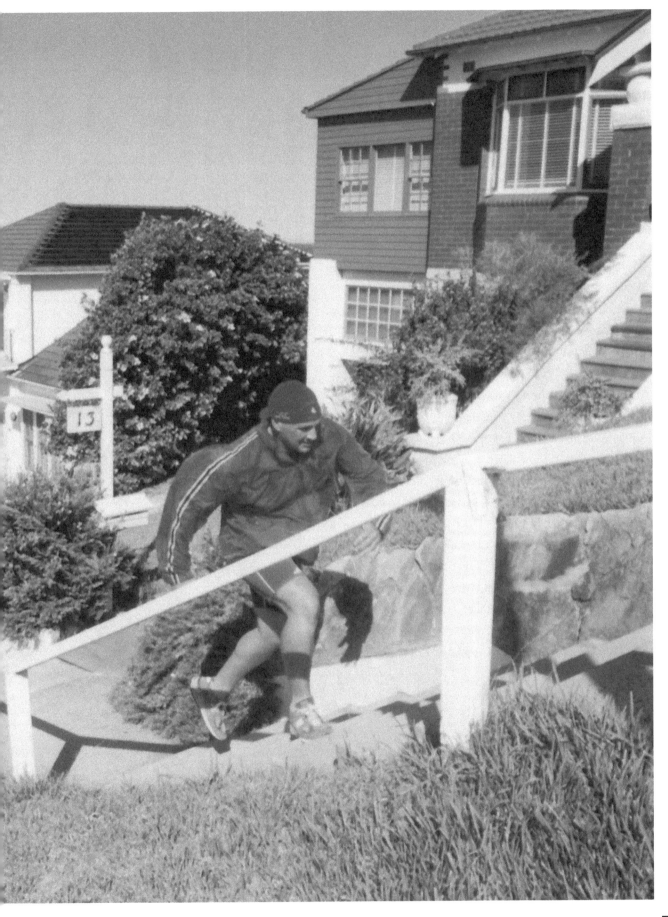

miles, but believe me, you shouldn't worry about the distance. All you should be interested in is the time you are out pounding the streets. Once you get into your own routine and you eventually work out a couple of different routes, you'll get familiar with the landscape of each route. Then you'll know when the hills are coming up and will be able to adjust your stride to suit. This will add a greater challenge to your run.

I have always included hills or steep stairs in my runs because it gives me more of a buzz when I finish. At first it will seem like a nightmare, especially when you approach the hill, but once you get to the top you'll have a great sense of achievement. Hey, was Rocky happy when he topped the steps? You bet he was! Don't worry if you have to stop — that happens to everyone. Just make a mental note of where you had to stop, and next time try to go a bit farther. Eventually, you'll get to the top without stopping and when you do it will feel great. It's a huge boost to your confidence.

Everyone is different, but when I get near the end of my run, I usually slow down to a jog, then I stop with about 100 meters to go and just walk the rest of the way. When I get to the finish, I check my stopwatch and repeat the stretching routine I started off with. I then go for a shower and have a nice cold drink (usually an isotonic drink or good old water). I have followed this routine through all my years of training. Even now when I beat a personal best or conquer another steep set of stairs, the buzz is still there, strong as ever. It's as good and intense a natural high as you can have.

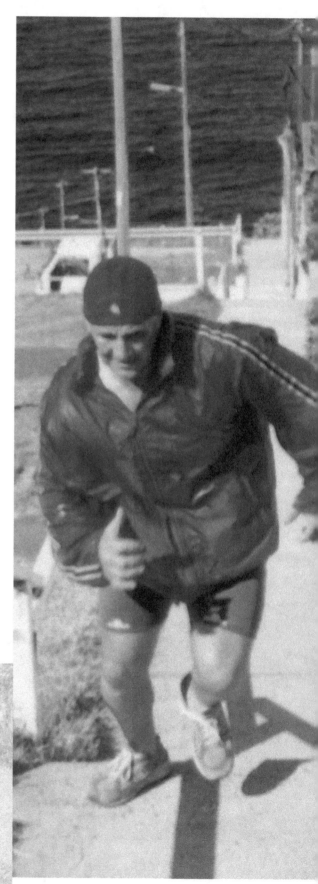

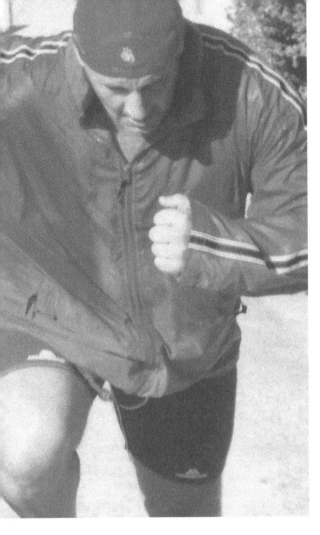

SPRiNTS

Sprinting, or explosive speed training, is another discipline that should be incorporated into your fitness program. The athletes in this book have all used speed work in their training camps. A typical speed training session might go like this:

1 Full body stretch (usual warm-up exercises for 10 minutes)
2 Jogging (for 5 minutes or, if you are training at an athletics track, 2 x 400 m laps at slow to medium pace)
3 Light stretching
4 100 meter sprint at full speed
5 1 minute rest
6 100 meter sprint at full speed
7 1 minute rest
8 Repeat 100 meter sprints and rest periods until you reach *your* maximum
9 Jogging (balance with your jogging warm-up — step 2)
10 Light stretching to finish

it's a well-known fact that Evander Holyfield hated running and preferred to work in the gym. When Lennox Lewis was about to fight Holyfield, he asked his trainer, Emanuel Steward, why he insisted that he do so much roadwork. Steward told him that he knew Holyfield wouldn't be doing any. You see, Steward had trained Holyfield for a lot of his big fights and he had to force him to run, sometimes even running with him to make sure he did it. Emanuel Steward was a smart cookie; he told Lewis this so that he would stop complaining about his grueling roadwork schedule and persevere. He also wanted to give Lewis a psychological edge in the remainder of their training camp.

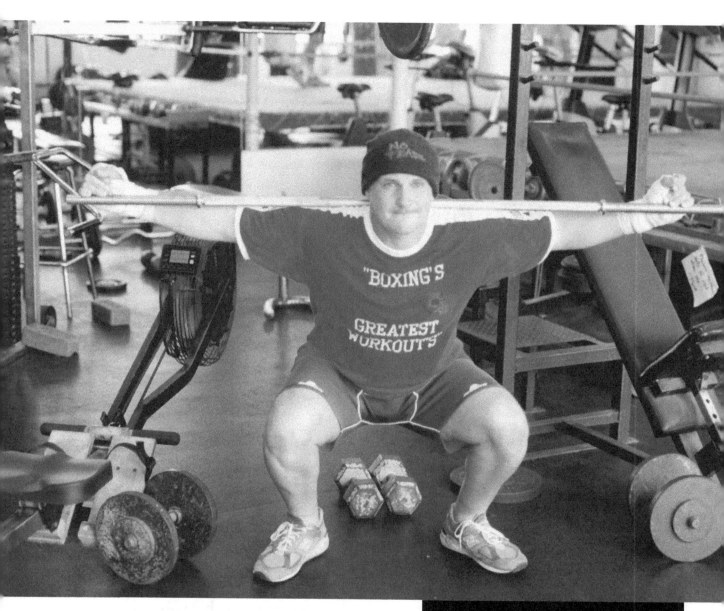

GYMWORK

Having a structured exercise regime is important, both physically and mentally. Gymwork is essential to my overall workout, so it makes sense to get the best possible results from it. Some people find it hard to stay focused in the gym. My tip: keep it fresh, mix it up, try new things and always look for new challenges. Speak to trainers, listen to their advice and use your own experience. For maximum benefit, be sure to integrate gymwork with roadwork. My program (*page 132*) suggests ways to do this effectively.

Leg squats

These are excellent for stretching the large, strong muscles in your hips and back. Keep your back straight and squat until you are comfortable. When you reach your limit, bounce up by pushing off your legs. Keep up a good pace until finished.

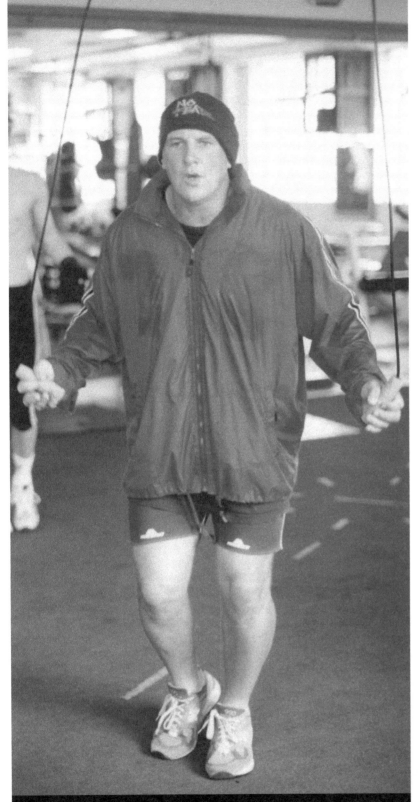

SIDE-TO-SIDES

Side-to-side stretching is a great way to loosen up before a run or your gymwork. Make sure you breathe normally and don't let your opposite shoulder drop forward.

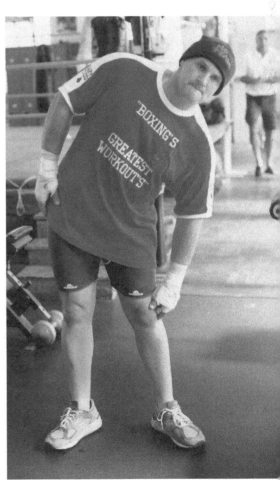

Jumping rope

If you're a beginner, or you're tripping up on the rope, try jumping on the spot without the rope, moving your hands and arms as if you have a rope. Start off slowly and pick a spot on the wall (or wherever suits you) and focus on it. This will give you something to build on. Gradually increase your time jumping rope as your fitness improves.

PUNCHiNG OUT

You can do this exercise with or
without hand weights. It's excellent
for warming up. Do it watching the
clock — this will actually help you.

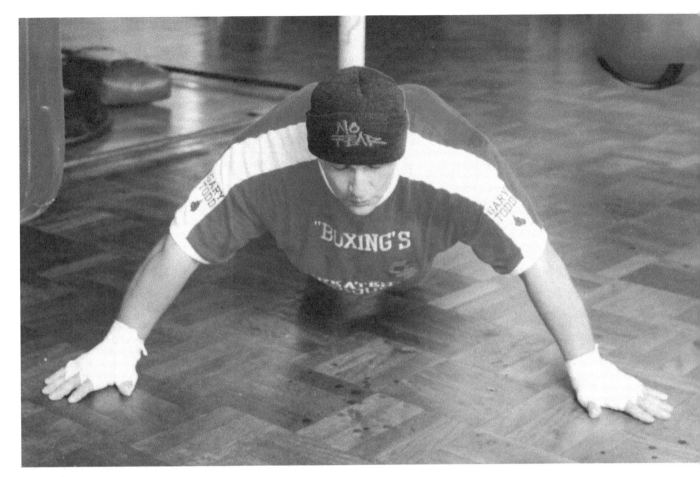

PUSH-UPS

A great way to increase upper-body strength. There are many ways to do push-ups and it's a good idea to include a variety in your workout. Here are just a few:

1 Put your hands flat on the floor, shoulder-width apart. Keep your back straight and lower your body until you touch the floor with your chest, then push yourself up again.

2 Put your hands flat on the floor as far apart as you can manage. Lower your body until you touch the floor with your chest, then push yourself up again.

3 Start as for No.1, but lift one leg and hold it straight while you lower your body and touch the floor with your chest. Push yourself up again and bring your leg back down. Do the next one lifting the other leg.

4 Start as for No.1, but when you push your body back up from the floor, spring or push your body up off the palms of your hands, clap hands, then put them back on the floor and lower your body again.

Touching toes

This is an important exercise to stretch your hamstrings. Make sure you keep your legs straight and hold for 10 seconds.

Torso twists

Torso twists help to warm up the spine. Be careful not to let your hips swing.

Arms swings

Great for warming up the shoulders and loosening up the shoulder joint. Remember: to get the benefit, brace you abs and don't arch your back.

SHADOWBOXING

Shadowboxing is all about coordination and working on your combinations. Always stay on your toes and bounce from one foot to the other. You don't have to go crazy: you are working on your combinations and punching techniques, not your power. Build up gradually and concentrate on your movements. If your gym has a mirror, then shadowbox in front of it. After you warm up, your arms and body should be hot and loose, but be careful not to over-punch or overextend your arms; this could cause injury to your elbow joints. Start slowly and pace yourself for your 3 minutes, building up speed as you go.

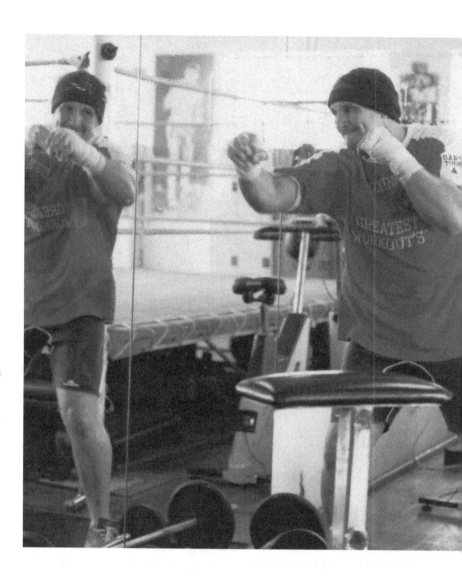

Heavy bag drilling

Before I start with my combinations routine on the bag, I drill the heavy bag to wake up my muscles. Punch at a fast and steady pace, pushing the bag forward as you go. Do not let the bag come back to you. I line up the bottom of the bag with a spot on the floor. Keep the bag in the same position and punch until your time is up. Do not watch the clock while you are on the heavy bag.

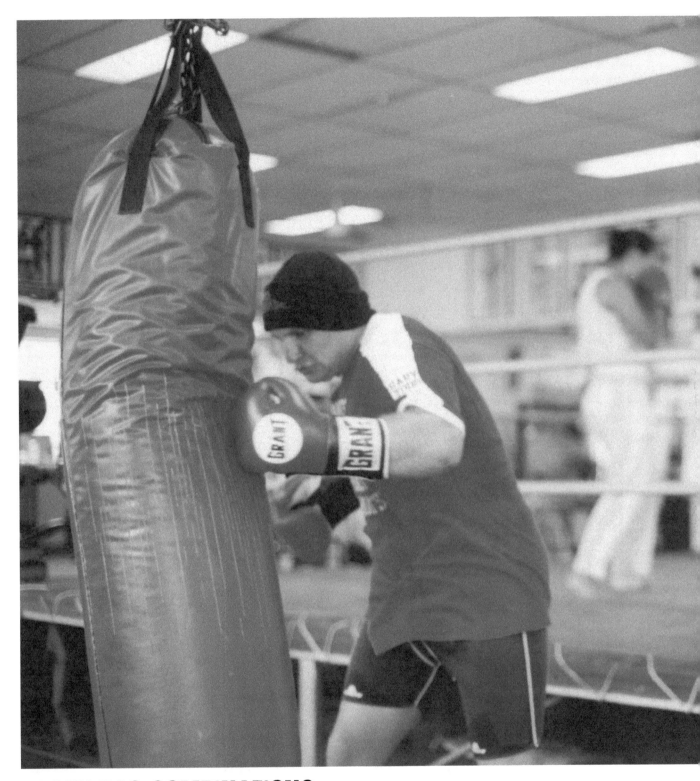

HEAVY BAG COMBINATIONS

Heavy bag work is extremely grueling, so you must pace yourself. If you go all-out in the first minute, then there's a good chance you'll burn out before your 3–5 minutes are up on the clock. Start off slowly and work on your footwork and combinations. Once you get your footwork going — moving in and out and pushing off your back foot — your punches will flow smoothly.

FOCUS PADS

Working on the pads is one of the most popular boxing exercises. This is where you can fine-tune combinations and try new and exciting punches with your trainer. Patience is important. You'll need to talk and listen to each other carefully and accept each other's mistakes. Create your own workout using suggestions from *My Program* (page 132).

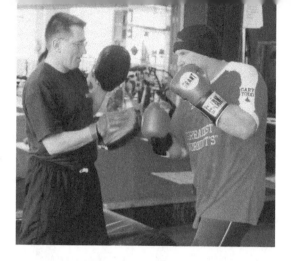

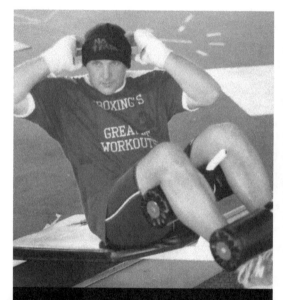

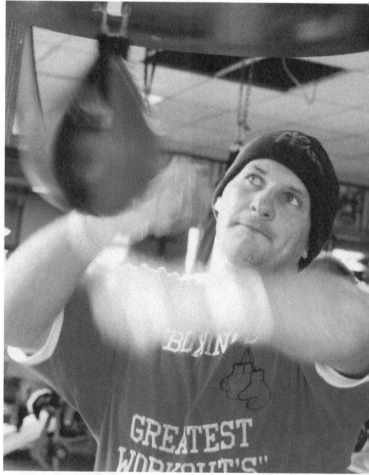

Abdominal exercises

There are many exercises for the abs, but these are the two I prefer. They're easy to perfect. Start off by getting positioned on a raised bench and getting your feet and bottom in a comfortable position.

1 Place your hands behind your head, or your fingertips on your temples, and sit up. As you sit up and let yourself back down again, be aware of your abs and make sure you are using them rather than straining your back.

2 Once you perfect the sit-up, try adding a twist as you come up, just touching your right knee with your left elbow, then your left knee with your right elbow.

SPEED BAG

This is a tricky piece of equipment but it can be mastered. It's all about patience and practice. Make sure the bottom of the bag is at your eye level. Start off with your left fist punching downward onto the ball. Once you achieve a steady drumming with your left, do exactly the same pace with your right fist. When you can do this with confidence, alternate and build up speed.

Leg-raises

Lie on your back and get as comfortable as you can. Use a mat if you have one. Place your hands on the floor at your sides and stretch out your legs, pointing your toes. All you have to do is lift your feet off the floor. There are different ways you can do leg-raises. Here are a few variations:

1 Lift your legs all the way up, then lower them back down until you just touch the floor for a moment, then lift them again and repeat.

2 Lift your feet (keeping your toes pointed) about 6 inches off the floor; hold for 1 minute.

3 Lift your feet (keeping your toes pointed) about 6 inches off the floor; hold for 30 seconds. Then cross one foot over the other, alternating which foot is on top for 30 seconds.

4 Lift one foot 6 inches off the floor, then lower it to the floor and lift the other foot. Continue lifting one foot then the other for 1 minute.

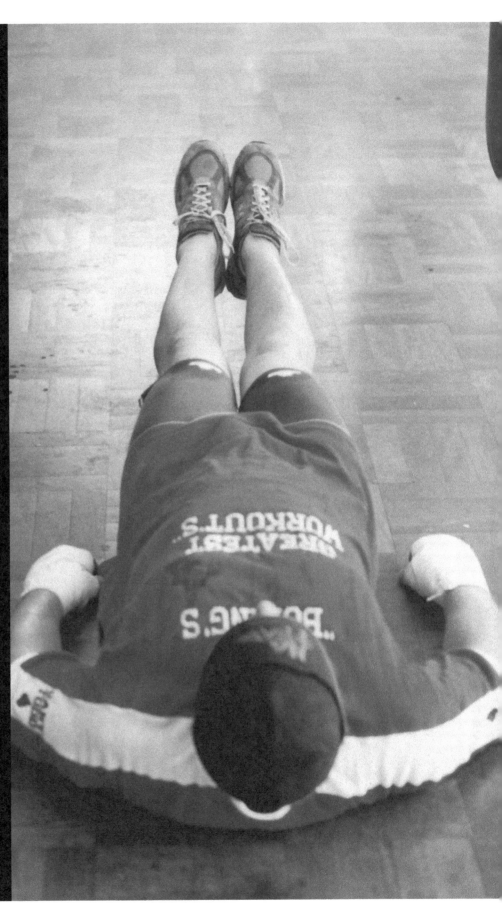

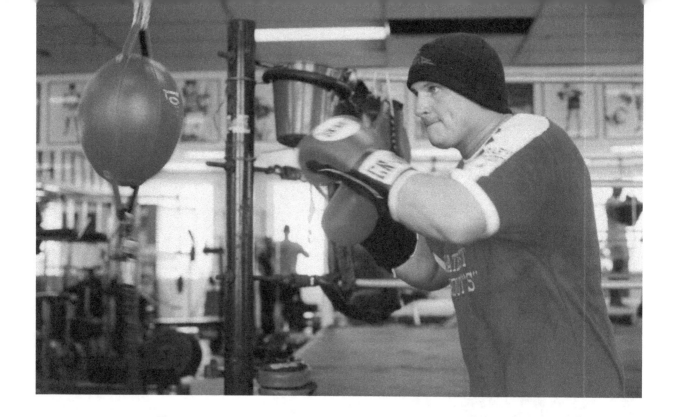

FLOOR-TO-CEiLiNG BAG

This exercise is all about reflexes and hand–eye coordination. Once you have found your range, start by trying one punch with the left hand then one with the right. Stay on your toes at all times and remember you don't have to punch hard. Test it by throwing a jab at the bag and see how far it comes back to you. Don't worry if the bag goes everywhere — that's what it's designed to do! Focus on the bag and be patient.

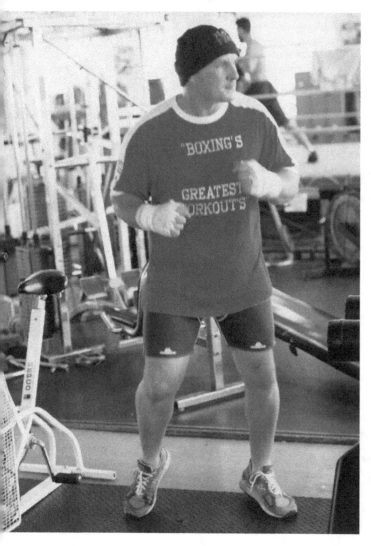

WARM DOWN

Jog on the spot, then bounce on your toes and move around. Keep your arms and shoulders loose. This is a good way to finish off your workout. Set your own time.

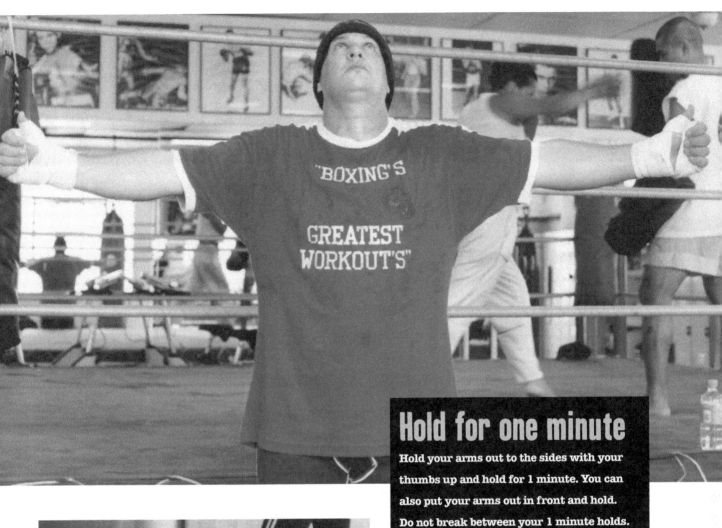

Hold for one minute

Hold your arms out to the sides with your thumbs up and hold for 1 minute. You can also put your arms out in front and hold. Do not break between your 1 minute holds.

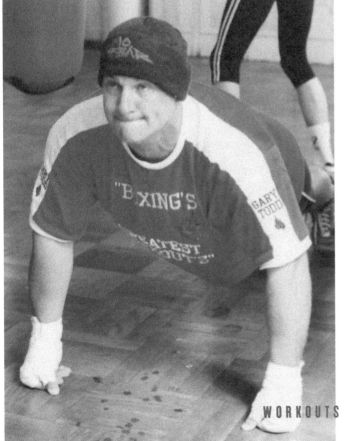

PUSHiNG iT HARD

Push-ups are a good way to finish off your workout. They also let you know how much strength you have left at the end. If you've pushed yourself to the limit, then you should be struggling with them. I like to do them on my knuckles.

MY PROGRAM

SIZE YOURSELF UP

i've arranged my program into beginner, intermediate and advanced levels, but you can tailor the number of reps, times and distances to your own needs as you get used to them. if you're unsure, start off at the beginner level. The following, however, is non-negotiable and extremely important: Consult a health professional before you begin any exercise or diet program, particularly if you're just starting out, you're over 35 or coming back from a long layoff.

WHAT LEVEL ARE YOU?

	Beginner	Intermediate	Advanced	
	You've been working out for less than six months.	You've been working out at least 3 or 4 times a week for the last six months.	You've been working out at least 5 to 6 times a week for the last 12 months, focusing on cardiovascular exercise.	
Action Plan				
Monday	Sprints	Jog/Run	Sprints	**Note:** If there's nothing in
Tuesday		Gym	Gym	the Intermediate or Advanced
Wednesday	Jog/Run		Jog/Run	columns in the following,
Thursday		Jog/Run	Gym	then assume the same as
Friday	Gym		Jog/Run	the Beginner level.
Saturday		Gym	Gym	
Sunday	Gym	Sprints		

warm-up

	Beginner	Intermediate	Advanced	
Touching toes	Hold for 10 seconds			Keep your legs straight and feel the stretch.
Hamstrings stretch	Hold for 10 seconds			Lift your left leg and rest your ankle at waist-height on a fence or wall or even on the back of your car. Try to put the fingertips of both hands on your toes. Repeat with the right leg.
Thigh stretch	Hold for 10 seconds			Pull your left leg up behind you and then pull your foot in toward your butt until you can feel the stretch. Repeat with the right leg.
Torso twists	50 each way	100 each way	150 each way	Stand up straight, lift your arms up to chest level with your hands or knuckles pointing in toward each other in front of your chest. Spread your legs slightly (more than shoulder-width) until you are balanced, then start to swivel your torso gently to the right. Stop for a split second, then swivel to the left. Keep your hips still.
Leg squats	10 reps			Stand up straight with your feet apart. Hold a broom handle or place your hands on your head. Bend your knees and squat down as low as you can go. Then bounce back up and continue at a steady pace.
Drink				

Sprints	Beginner	Intermediate	Advanced
Jog	5 min. If you're training at an athletics track, 2 x 400 meter laps, slow to medium pace		
Light stretching	Hamstrings, calves, groin		
Sprints	3 x 20 meter (20 sec. rest between sprints)	5 x 20 meter	7 x 20 meter
Rest & drink	1 min.		
Sprints	3 x 40 meter (20 sec. rest between sprints)	5 x 40 meter	7 x 40 meter
Rest & drink	1 min.		
Sprints	3 x 60 meter (20 sec. rest between sprints)	5 x 60 meter	7 x 60 meter
Rest & drink	1 min.		
Sprints	1 x 100 meter		
Jog	5 min. slow jog, as per warm-up		
Drink			

Jog/Run	Beginner	Intermediate	Advanced
Warm-up	As for sprints		
Run	25 min.	30 min., ending with a hill or a sprint	40 min., ending with a hill or a sprint
Warm-down	Light stretching as per warm-up		

Gymwork	Beginner	Intermediate	Advanced	
Warm-up				
Touching toes	Hold for 10 seconds			Keep your legs straight and feel the stretch.
Torso twists	30 each way	40 each way	50 each way	Refer to **Roadwork** section for instruction.
Side-to-sides	30 each side	40 each side	50 each side	Stand with your feet about a foot apart, your arms by your sides and your palms on your thighs. Tilt your upper body to the left, letting your hand slide down your thigh until it touches the side of your knee. Straighten up and repeat to the right. Don't let opposite shoulder drop forward.
Arm swings	30 each side	40 each side	50 each side	Start with your palms on the top of your thighs. Swing one arm up above your head and back as far as you can, while you swing the other behind you as far as you can. Alternate one arm up and one down.
Leg squats	10 reps	20 reps	30 reps	Refer to **Roadwork** section for instruction.
Punching out	3 x 1 min. rounds (30 sec. break after each round)	3 x 2 min. (with or without hand weights)	3 x 3 min. (with hand weights)	With your arms at chest level punch straight out.
Jumping rope	3 min.	4 min.	5 min.	Start at moderate pace until you get into your own groove. Pick a spot on the wall and focus on it, or if there's a mirror, jump in front of it. As you improve, try and move to and fro.

Note: Right after you finish jumping rope, it's time to get your hand wraps on. Some people put their wraps on before they start jumping rope, but I like to do it after.

Gymwork	Beginner	Intermediate	Advanced	
Push-ups	15 reps	25 reps	40 reps	Any of the four push-ups suggested on page 125.
Main Set				
Shadowboxing	3 x 3 min. rounds (60 sec. break after each round)	3 x 3 min. (45 sec. break)	3 x 3 min. (30 sec. break)	Start by standing with your left leg forward and your right leg behind. Bounce up and around and get your feet stable. Then lift your hands up to your chin and flick out your left hand in a slow-motion movement. Follow up with a straight right hand.
Heavy bag drilling (Alternate with focus pads)	3 x 3 min. rounds, working on combinations (30 sec. break after each round)	3 x 4 min.	3 x 5 min.	Start with your hands up at chest level and stand with your knees slightly bent. Punch out and upward, drilling the bag at a fast, steady pace, pushing the bag forward as you go.
Heavy bag combinations	3 x 3 min. rounds, working on combinations (30 sec. break after each round)	3 x 4 min.	3 x 5 min.	Focus on your footwork first, then your punches. Start off slowly, working on your combinations. Move in and out, pushing off your back foot. "Snap" your punches out and in, bringing your hands back to the side of your head.
Floor-to-ceiling bag	5 min. (1 min. break)	7.5 min.	10 min.	Find your range. Test this by throwing a jab at the bag and see how far it comes back to you. Stay on your toes. Try one punch with the left hand, then one with the right until you get a feel for it. As your control develops, try doubling up on your jab and incorporate left and right hooks. In time, you'll start throwing combinations.

Gymwork	Beginner	Intermediate	Advanced	
Focus pads (If you don't have someone to hold the pads for you, substitute with heavy bag)	3 x 1 min. rounds, working on combinations (30 sec. break after each round)	3 x 2 min.	3 x 3 min.	Create your own program. Start by counting out uppercuts in groups of 2, 4, 6, up to 20, and then back down to 2. You can jumble the numbers around, or you can go by the clock.
Sit-ups	3 x 20 (30 sec. break after each set)	3 x 35	3 x 50	Refer to page 128 for instructions.
Leg-raises	3 x 10 reps (30 sec. break after each set)	3 x 15 reps	3 x 20 reps	Refer to page 129 for instructions.
Speed bag	3 min. (followed by a 1 min. break)	4 min.	5 min.	Make sure you get the height right. The bottom of the bag should be at eye level. If it's too high, put a couple of barbell plates on the floor and stand on them. Refer to page 128 for instructions.
Drink (and take off your hand wraps)				
Warm-down, jogging in place	2 min.	2 min.	2 min.	
Light stretching, bouncing around on toes	2 min.	2 min.	2 min.	
Hold for 1 min	Hold your arms out to the side, thumbs up, for 1 min.			
Push-ups	15	20	25 on knuckles	

Drink, shower

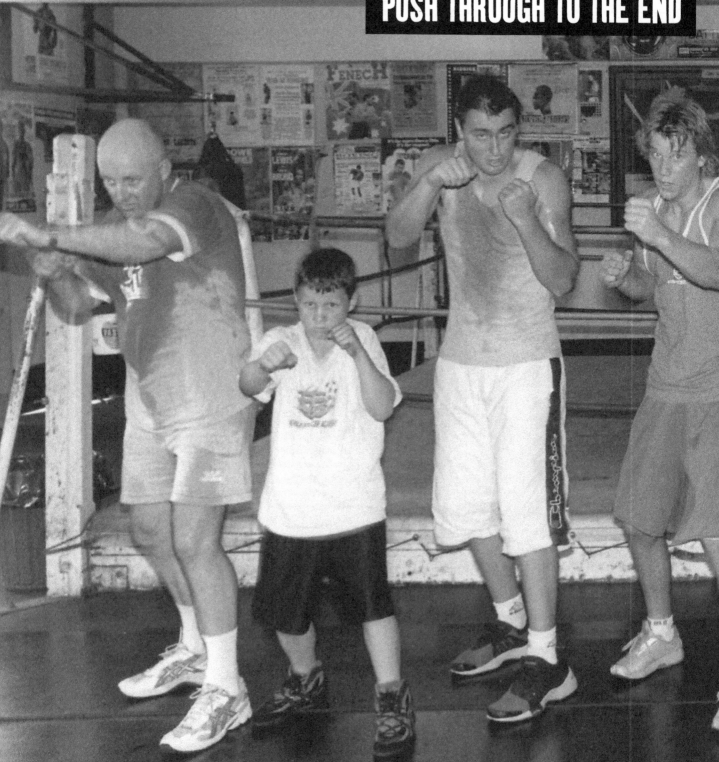

WORK HARD, TRAIN HARD

BE YOUR BEST

PUSH THROUGH TO THE END

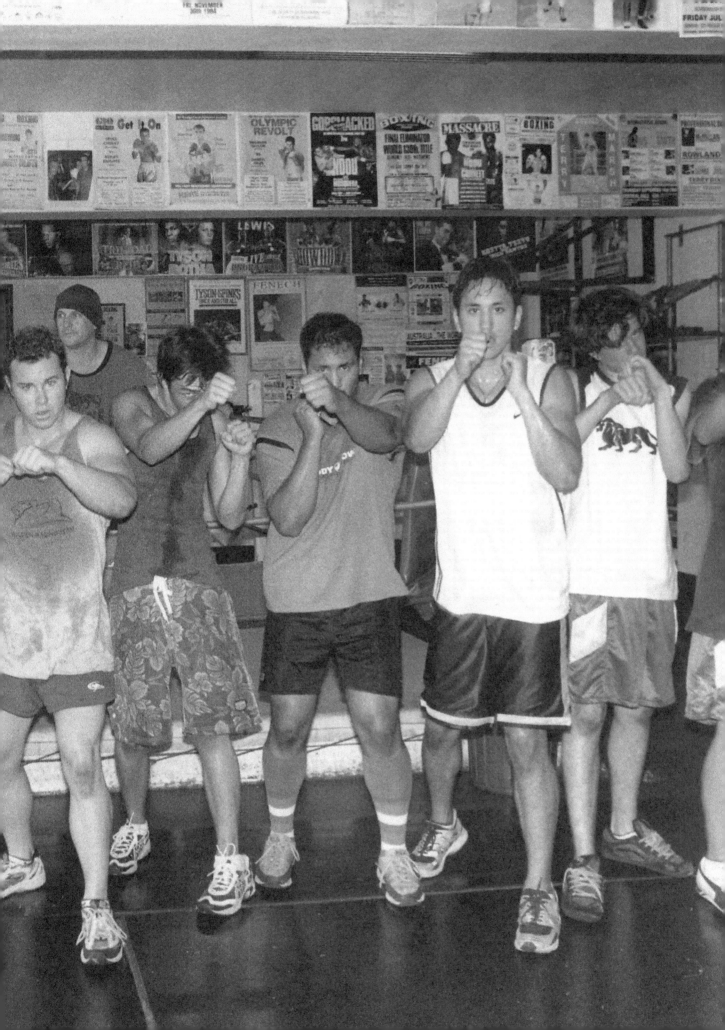

WHEN i MET...

i've traveled the world to watch and learn from my heroes. i just soak up the atmosphere and have a great time doing it. Here are some memories from a self-confessed boxaholic's travels. it's a hard job ... but someone's got to do it!

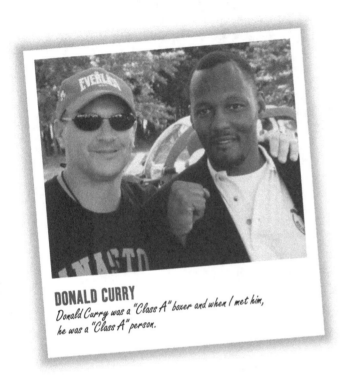

DONALD CURRY
Donald Curry was a "Class A" boxer and when I met him, he was a "Class A" person.

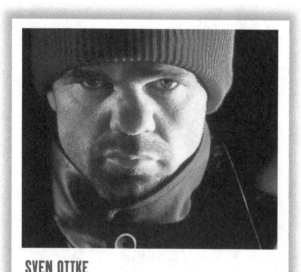

SVEN OTTKE
I interviewed Sven through an interpreter, but he was very patient and was as classy as they come.

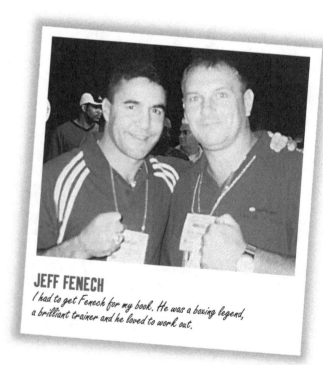

JEFF FENECH
I had to get Fenech for my book. He was a boxing legend, a brilliant trainer and he loved to work out.

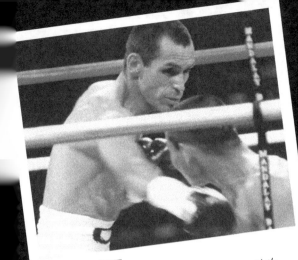

RICARDO LOPEZ

I met Ricardo in New York and the interview was done with the help of a translator. It was a long interview, but it was worth it. A true gentleman.

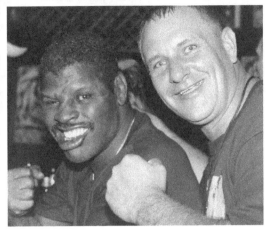

LEON SPINKS

Spinks was a challenge to interview. He couldn't understand my Dundee accent – and I couldn't understand him. What a laugh!

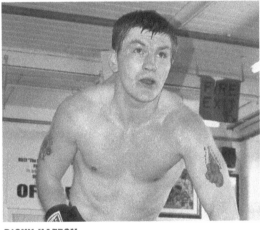

RICKY HATTON

Hatton is the most exciting boxer to come out of Britain since Nigel Benn. He never takes a backward step. He trains intensely in camp and uses his conditioning to overwhelm his opponents in the ring.

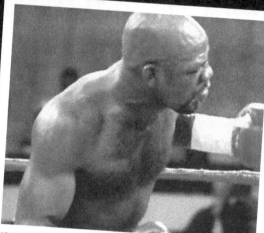

IRAN BARKLEY

I met Iran Barkley in the "Gracianos" bar in Canastota, New York. It was late. We had a few drinks and a long chat together. A good guy.

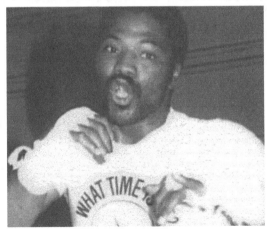

AARON PRYOR

I met Aaron in New York and he was a dream to interview. He's a complete gentleman.

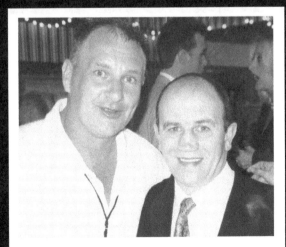

CHARLIE MAGRI

Charlie Magri is the most down-to-earth boxer I've ever met and a true champion.

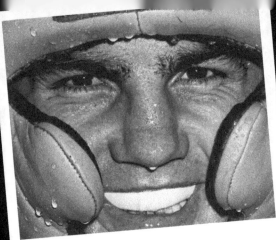

JEFF HARDING
Harding was a tough, hard boxer. He gave his all for himself and his country.

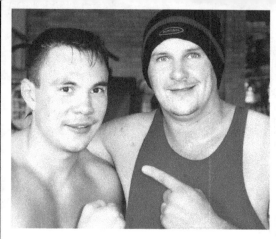

KOSTYA TSZYU
When I watched Tszyu in the gym, it was unbelievable. I said, "Well done, Kostya," and he said, "Zat vos nussink. I can do better!"

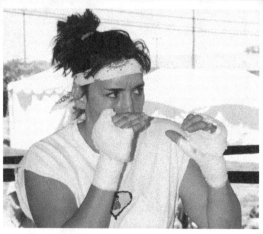

CHRISTY MARTIN
Christy showed the determination and courage to become the Number One in women's boxing around the world.

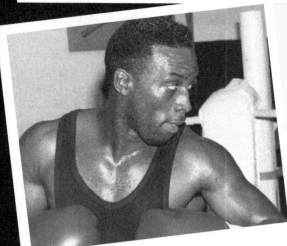

NIGEL BENN
Benn was the most exciting fighter in the gym. When you were around him, there was an indescribable aura. A really intense trainer.

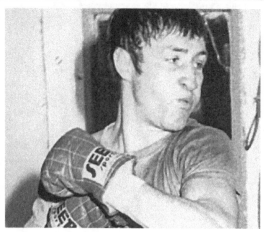

KEN BUCHANAN
Ken Buchanan was a brilliant and dedicated boxer who didn't take any shortcuts. He fought the best boxers in their own backyards and won.

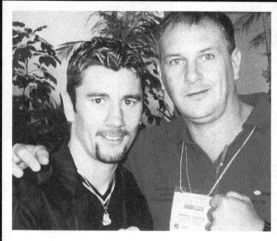

WAYNE MCCULLOUGH
Wayne McCullough is pure class, in and out of the ring.

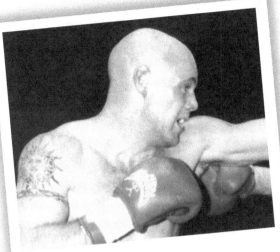

GLENN CATLEY
Catley gives his all in the gym and he was a pleasure to interview.

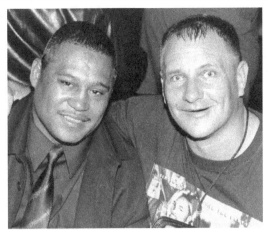

JUAN LAPORTE
LaPorte was quite serious when I interviewed him. He was due to fight "The Professor," Azumah Nelson, so I suppose that was understandable. Good boxer, good guy.

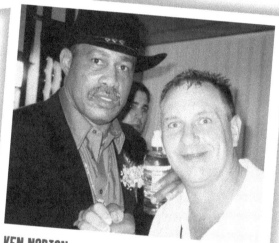

KEN NORTON
Ken Norton was a "hard-as-nails" boxer in the ring, but a kind, gentle man outside the ring. Training was his life.

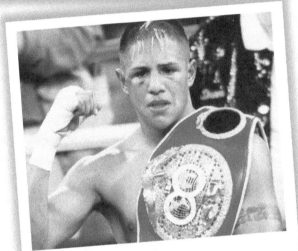

FERNANDO VARGAS
I interviewed Fernando at the weigh-in at Madison Square Garden. I walked up to him and he growled at me.

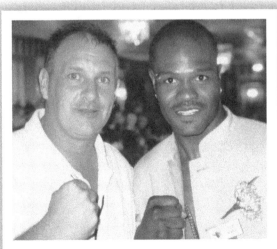

MUHAMMAD ALI
To get to Ali, I had to get past his bodyguards. I annoyed them so much that they gave me five minutes. Five minutes lasted 20. It was an unforgettable experience.

TERRY NORRIS
Norris was a charming, softly spoken man and was a pleasure to talk to.

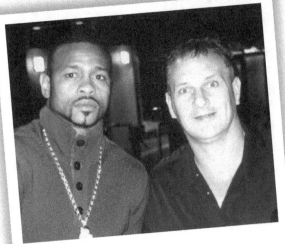

ROY JONES JUNIOR
People say a lot of things about Jones Junior, but most of the time he leaves people speechless.

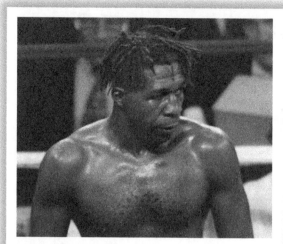

LIVINGSTONE BRAMBLE
Livingstone Bramble was the happiest and most talkative boxer I interviewed. He was great company.

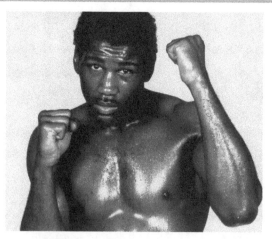

MATTHEW SAAD MUHAMMAD
Saad Muhammad was a great fighter and loved to work out in the gym. Always strong and fit.

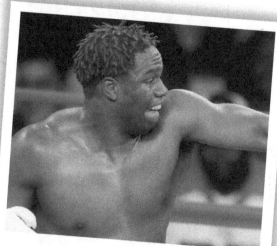

CHRIS BYRD
Good guy, great boxer.

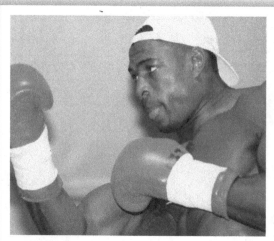

FRANK BRUNO
I met Frank in Las Vegas, just before the Tyson fight. I thought to myself, "This guy deserves to win the world title." What a trainer in the gym!

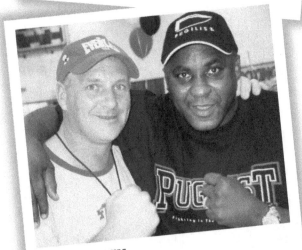

MIKE MCCALLUM
It took me three days to get him to do the interview. He was always fooling around. I didn't care, because it was three days with a legend.